"The book is a great resource, providing inforr affected by mental health issues during the per can have on all of those involved during this ir all types of ways that mental health issues can manifest and offers some great advice too. Thanks to Jane and Mark for getting this book together; it will be so beneficial to many"

Ashley Curry, volunteer for OCD Action and Maternal OCD,
keynote speaker for the NHS and the Maternal Mental Health Alliance,
lay member and researcher for Tourette's Action
and teacher of IAPT therapists for OCD.

"This timely book arrives when the place of men in Western society is poorly defined and less secure. Driven by post-industrial economics, the role of the woman, Dr Hanley and Mr Williams suggest, has been recast as both bread-winner and mother, leaving the male partner excluded and vulnerable. These changes, they claim, lead to mental health problems for the entire family but most perniciously for fathers. Controversially, they propose a surprising champion for the status quo"

Stephen Paul Jones, RMN, BA, MBA,
retired lecturer in Mental Health Nursing.

"This exceptional book by Mark Williams and Dr Jane Hanley is likely to quickly become the go-to resource for fathers' mental health. Written expertly and sensitively, it covers everything we need to know about diagnoses and conditions, the impact on the whole family, infant bonding and interaction, and crucial information on treatment and management. This book will shatter the stigma that fathers face and help make it more likely that they will come forward to get the support they need."

Dr Andrew Mayers, perinatal mental health expert,
Bournemouth University.

Fathers and Perinatal Mental Health

It is only in recent years that there has been development in the awareness of the father's mental health. Yet, the father's mental health can influence the mother, the infant, the family and society. This book seeks to address the reasons why the father or the potential father could suffer from a mental disorder or illness during the perinatal period, his reactions and what can be done to help him.

The book explores the way in which a father's mental health has presented in the past and how it presents now. It looks at the father's attitudes towards his mental well-being and how he may self-manage and self-medicate. It examines the impact and influence the potential father and the father's mental health has on his partner, infant and children. The reasons for certain disorders and illnesses are outlined, along with how they may manifest and are managed. Treatment options and types of medication are discussed and the ways in which the father can access the best possible help and support. Stories from fathers who have suffered from a particular mental illness or condition help others to understand both the practicalities and realities.

The uniqueness of the shared stories from fathers highlights why recognition, treatment and management are important to help other fathers improve their relationship with their partner and infant and to improve their own well-being. The book is intended to help health practitioners and anyone who is concerned about fathers' mental health.

Jane Hanley has had an interest in perinatal mental health for almost forty years. She has written, trained and lectured extensively on maternal and paternal mental health, both nationally and internationally. Jane has had two other books published on perinatal mental health.

Mark Williams is an author, speaker and international campaigner. In 2004 he himself experienced depression and anxiety after his son was born and has enhanced his knowledge after speaking to hundreds of parents since 2011. He has spoken on television and radio stations around the world and co-founded 'International Father's Mental Health Day'.

Fathers and Perinatal Mental Health

A Guide for Recognition, Treatment and Management

Jane Hanley and Mark Williams

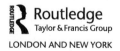
Routledge
Taylor & Francis Group

LONDON AND NEW YORK

First published 2020
by Routledge
2 Park Square, Milton Park, Abingdon, Oxon OX14 4RN

and by Routledge
52 Vanderbilt Avenue, New York, NY 10017

Routledge is an imprint of the Taylor & Francis Group, an informa business

British Library Cataloguing-in-Publication Data
A catalogue record for this book is available from the British Library

Library of Congress Cataloging-in-Publication Data
A catalog record has been requested for this book

ISBN: 978-1-138-33030-6 (hbk)
ISBN: 978-1-138-33032-0 (pbk)
ISBN: 978-0-429-44794-5 (ebk)

Typeset in Times New Roman
by Nova Techset Private Limited, Bengaluru & Chennai, India

Contents

Chapter 1

Fathers and perinatal mental health

Introduction

The state of being a father has changed, fatherhood has changed. The nuclear family with a mother, father and infant is no longer the norm (Ivens 2010). The past 20 years have seen changes in the average family unit. There are now more single fathers, same sex fathers and stay at home fathers with shared parenting. The diversity of situations has meant that society needs to take the concerns of fathers seriously. They are just as prone to suffer from mental illness in the perinatal period, as mothers. They can have attachment issues with their offspring and relationship difficulties with their partners. It is important that these factors are recognized, not only for the sake of the father, but for the sake of the family.

For a while now, the focus has been on the mental health of the mother during the perinatal period, and as a consequence, that includes the mental health of the infant. However, this was not always the case. For centuries, mothers with mental health 'problems' were either ignored by society or incarcerated into institutions. The literature is littered with mad women whose behaviour was so outside the norm following the birth of their baby, there was little chance they would be able to look after their infant, and more likely, would have both themselves and their child taken into some form of care (Brontë 1847, Gilbert & Gubar 1979).

If a woman became pregnant out of wedlock, that was always her fault and very little, if any, blame was laid on the man. In marriage, however, one of the prime responsibilities of the woman was to produce a son and heir. Matrimony was supposed to provide the safe haven in which to rear the child. The support of two parents, one to provide the childcare and the other to finance the arrangement was often the accepted convention. If fathers were mad, bad or indifferent, there were few who would challenge them. In the patriarchal societies, a social system where men held the primary power both within the home and in society, the man had the right to come and go as he pleased, with little to question his integrity or morals.

Madness and insanity were rarely talked about and often feared. The fear was borne out of ignorance and the inability to treat, and in some instances, cure the person. Men who were mentally ill with mania were ordinarily aggressive, abusive and difficult to contain. Those who suffered from depression were morose and self-deprecating, often with little thought for family and friends. Usually it was a one size fits all, with sparse definition of the differing types of mental illness. This differed from physical illnesses, which were clearly categorised and defined and yet mental illnesses were probably as complex and diverse; however, there remains confusion about the causes and courses.

Past history of mental health disorders

As discussions around father's mental health are recent, it is unlikely that the incidence would have been recorded in history. In fact, there is little historical reference to the relationship between mentally ill fathers and their children. Some of the more famous men who suffered from anxiety and depression had several children and included Charles Dickens, who had ten children as did Charles Darwin, Robert Schumann, who had had eight and President Lincoln who had four. Yet the information on their connections and bonding experiences with their offspring is sparse (Berra 2013).

History, however, suggests that the fathers who appeared to have suffered from mental disorders sometimes led miserable lives, with torn marriages and damaged relationships. This is illustrated in the works by Thornton (2008), who described how Graham Green, regarded as one of the greatest writers of the 20th century, had a history of bipolar disorder, which not only had a profound effect on, but influenced both his writing and his personal life. He had several sexual encounters during his marriage and was eventually estranged from his wife and children.

The effects of male depression are reiterated by Shenk (2005) who described the bouts of melancholy suffered by President Abraham Lincoln (1805–1865). The President experienced 'mental breakdowns' from his mid-thirties, where he regularly cried in public. He often described his feelings of hopelessness, being fatigued and frequently expressed suicidal thoughts.

Some, like the psychoanalyst and neurologist Sigmund Freud (1856–1939), who suffered from anxiety and depression, resorted to self-medicating by taking illicit drugs. Initially Freud consumed cocaine in small doses, and found that it made a significant difference to his mental health; however, he recognised its addictive qualities and in later life tended to thrive on the fact that the brilliance of his work was recognised (Jones 1975).

Although the father's features of 'madness' were known to the public, it appeared that their condition had to reach a crisis point before it was treated, when they were either admitted or incarcerated into an asylum, where the actual type of treatment was relatively unknown.

Writings by Steinberg (2016) suggested that Robert Schumann, regarded as one of the greatest German composers, suffered from severe 'melancholic depressive' episodes, alternating with phases of 'exaltation' which recurred several times during his short lifetime. He was also delusional and paranoid. When he attempted suicide at the age of fifty-four years, he self-referred to an asylum, where he was diagnosed with psychotic melancholia He remained there until his death two years later.

Edvard Munch, famously known for his painting 'The Scream', struggled with depression, anxiety, hallucinations, paranoia and alcoholism which were exacerbated by his drinking and fighting. He was known for his violent relationships with women. Munch admitted that he was able to relate his feelings of anxiety and depression to inform his expressionist art. He described his inspiration to paint 'The Scream' as … '*I stood there trembling with fear and felt how a long unending scream was going through the whole of nature*' (Faerna 1995, Prideaux 2005). His illness necessitated almost a year of therapy in a 'clinic'.

There are indications that mental illness could have a family history, as illustrated by President Abraham Lincoln, whose parents were both disposed to melancholy (Shenk 2005), whilst Munch's and Schumann's families' history of mental illness is well documented.

The artists who reached public attention and fame because of their art, writings or music were inspired, in the most part, by their mental illnesses and felt their conditions enhanced their artistic capabilities. Naifeh and Smith (2011) described Van Gogh as '*a quintessential, misunderstood genius where madness and creativity converged*', a term which could easily describe some of the other artists. However, it is suspected that this does not include the less famous or less fortunate men, whose histories of mental illness are unrecorded, but form part of the narratives of families. There is often a reluctance to discuss those who were termed 'mad' or 'deranged' and who may have resorted to the abuse of alcohol and women to qualm their unruly thoughts and behaviours.

Asylums

This litany of historical facts highlights that mental illness has always been a feature of mankind, yet begs the question if science has really progressed in the bid to find a cure. The days of the asylum have long disappeared, because of the negative effects involved in the process of institutionalisation. This, despite the fact that the complete withdrawal from society, to include no contact with friends or family and no reminders of anything that would aggravate the mind did not accelerate a cure. This was found to be a therapeutic method to alleviate the madness. There are numerous therapeutic interventions available which imitate those offered in the asylums and include having the opportunity to convene with nature, taking long walks, becoming active and socialising with those of a like mind (Evans 2018).

Men are no longer incarcerated, but they are still locked up 'for their and the safety of others', in a jail, if they display aggressive antisocial behaviour. It is often the police force that responds and takes control of a situation where a man suffering from hostile hallucinations, reacts to them or the man who walks into the sea, because he is determined to end his depressed, miserable life. Frequently, it is the police who are first on the scene of a suicide. Many are known to the mental health services and the recognition of the lack of available, suitable beds means they are often 'released' into a community that cannot provide the respite, rest and recuperation that they need. The importance of a safe and stable environment in which to live and work cannot be overstated. The statistics suggest that men are over ten times more likely to commit suicide than women. There are approximately eighty-four deaths in the UK by suicide every week. Depressed men are more likely to be suicidal than those with no low mood disorder.

Asylums have been replaced with community units and crisis teams. However, the polarisation of the debate between hospital and community care has moved on, and the development of mental health crisis and home teams, assertive outreach and early intervention teams has improved mental health services. The debate about the amount of monies needed for services is constant, with successive governments promising ever larger amounts. However, as with all promises, the total is never enough to cater to the needs of a population, which is reaching a crisis in poor mental health.

Present day management

Today, therapy, if available, is offered, but men are notoriously reluctant to accept 'talking therapies' because of its stigmatising effect, and the impact of admitting to a stranger that they are unable to cope with their relationships, job and self. This is slowly changing, and there have been significant advances in the opportunities for men to talk freely about how they feel. Prominent members of public and royalty have freely expressed how they have and have not coped with their personal demons. This is evidenced by the honest stories throughout this book which highlight how men were unable to cope and if they were lucky enough, how therapy helped them to progress and attain happy relationships with their partner, infant and family.

However, there are limitations to the types of therapy that can be accessed and often it includes taking antidepressants. The bad press around the long-term effects of the medication can deter men from taking them, particularly when they experience the disabling side effects which may impact their libido. Many resort to self-medication by abusing drugs because of the instant 'fix' it has to relieve their pain, yet many are ignorant of the damage alcohol and drugs can do to their mental health. Both exacerbate their symptoms of anxiety and depression, including the harmful effects on the brain circuitry, generating thoughts of paranoia and experiences of hallucinations and delusions.

Misusing alcohol, a familiar historical trait, is also deleterious to mental health, yet is often seen as the most efficient way of managing stress and anxiety, as well as perking up low mood. Alcohol, however, can be a destructive force and as history shows, has the propensity to devastate families and relationships. The demise of the public house, many of which were forced to close because of smoking and drunk driving laws, has disadvantaged the man who used to share a pint with fellow drinkers and now prefers, or rather is used to, drinking the cheaper alcohol sold in the supermarket. Smoking tobacco, although not as common as abusing alcohol, is taken to alleviate stress, but has the same harmful properties which can affect not only the physical but mental health.

Purging toxins was a common occurrence and the use of laxatives and enemas were used to release them from the digestive system. Traditionally the diet was important for mental health, and it was thought that toxic substances which built up in the body needed to be released. Today emetics are used to lose weight but not strictly for health reasons, but to maintain body dysmorphia, in an effort to combat anxiety. Over indulging in the fat-filled fast food diets, which with their high sugar content, offer instant release from misery and the consequences, not only destroy physical health but there is a penalty for their mental health.

As society becomes enslaved by the blue light screens of phones and iPads, the habit of sleep and rest is diminished. Sleep has a profound impact on mental health. The circadian rhythms of sleep have a significant influence on mental health and dictate how we generally feel. Poor sleep patterns exacerbate depressive symptoms and inadequate sleep can precipitate mental illness. Despite this knowledge, reports suggest that society is now in a constant state of 'work' stress, with access to information technology twenty-four hours a day, and sleep hygiene is dictated by this technology.

All of this would be irrelevant if mental health were not the most important health, 'No health without mental health' (DHSS 2011). At last society has taken note of the mental health of mothers-to-be and mothers. There is a myriad of evidence, research and studies which catalogue the types of mental illness. Work is progressing on epigenetics and neuroscience and the impact this has on motherhood. There is increasing skill in assessment techniques and with a sound knowledge of their capabilities and limitations, health practitioners are able to treat, manage or refer on mothers with a mental illness or disorder.

The mental health of the infant has been studied and the hazards in utero are established. There is now a sound grasp on the development of the foetal brain and the importance of nurturing. The issues around behaviour and attachment are well documented and health practitioners have the skills to help the mother and her infant bond.

The mental health of fathers, however, has been sadly neglected. Studies are emerging, and there is more thought on the role of the man as an integral part of the family, as a partner, and importantly as a father. Fathers feel somewhat disenfranchised from health services and often during the perinatal period, are omitted from the care of their partner and infant (Baldwin et al. 2018).

The awareness of the father's role and his transition to fatherhood is gaining momentum. This has been evidenced in the UK Government's 'Shared Parenting Leave' and the Health Service recognising some of the necessary provisions for fathers. There are, however, areas that require improvement which centre around of the inclusion the father during the antenatal period, an appreciation of his role in the Labour Ward, the importance of recognizing his stress in the Neonatal Unit, his involvement in the home visits and the importance of his part in infant attachment. There is, however, little recognition of the father's mental health, and to date, no formal assessment process.

Yet fathers can have mental ill health too and as the research suggests, the infant born to a depressed or anxious mother may, as a result, also suffer from anxiety and depression. Therefore, it makes sense that the father may have an ignored mental illness, which impacts his relationships. It is fortuitous that society is now beginning to recognise this, by attempting to make the perinatal period a time to research into why, when, where and how we can eradicate, or at least alleviate, mental illness for good. Good mental health is important for everyday living and no-one should suffer from poor mental health.

References

Baldwin S, Malone M, Sandall J, Bick D. 2018. Mental health and wellbeing during the transition to fatherhood: A systematic review of first time fathers' experiences. *JBI Database of System Reviews and Implementation Report*, 16(11), pp. 2118–2191.

Berra T. 2013. *Darwin and His Children. His Other Legacy.* New York: Oxford University Press.

Brontë C. 1847. *Jane Eyre.* London, UK: Penguin Classics.

DHSS. 2011. *No Health Without Mental Health: A Cross-Government Mental Health Outcomes Strategy for People of All Ages.* Gov.UK. https://www.google.com/search?q=DHSS.+2011.+No+Health+Without+Mental+Health%3A+A+Cross-Government+Mental+Health+Outcomes+Strategy+for+People+of+All+Ages.+Gov.UK.&rlz=1C1NHXL_enIN807IN807&oq=DHSS.+2011.+No+Health+Without+Mental+Health%3A+A+Cross-Government+Mental+Health+Outcomes+Strategy+for+People+of+All+Ages.+Gov.UK.&aqs=chrome..69i57.374j0j7&sourceid=chrome&ie=UTF-8, accessed 19 November 2019.

Evans E. 2018. *Mental Health Nursing.* A Personal Account. pp. 64–68. Some of the information is featured in the book: Carradice P, Goffin B (eds) 2014. *Behind Many Doors.* London, UK: Accent Press Ltd.

Faerna JM. 1995. *Munch.* New York, NY: Harry N. Abrahams, p. 16.

Gilbert S, Gubar S. 1979. *The Mad Woman in the Attic.* New Haven, CT: Yale University Press.

Ivens T. 2010. *Fatherhood in the 21st Century.* Carmarthen: UK Fatherskills Ltd.

Jones E. 1975. *The Life and Work of Sigmund Freud.* New York: Basic Books.

Naifeh SW, Smith GW. 2011. *Van Gogh: The Life.* New York: Random House.

Prideaux S. 2005. *Edvard Munch: Behind the Scream.* New Haven, CT: Yale University.

Shenk J. 2005. *Lincoln's Melancholy: How Depression Challenged a President and Fuelled His Greatness.* Boston, MA: Houghton Mifflin Harcourt.

Steinberg R. 2016. Robert Schumann in Endenich: The diagnosis and course of his illness and his illness-related experiences. *Journal of Community Medicine & Health Education*, 6, p. 466. doi:10.4172/2161-0711.1000466.

Thornton M. 2008. The decadent world of Graham Green – The high priest of darkness. *Daily Mail*, 19th March. https://www.dailymail.co.uk/news/article-539011/The-decadent-world-Graham-Greene--high-priest-darkness.html, accessed 18 October 2019.

Chapter 2

Importance of good perinatal mental health

Over the past five years it is being increasingly recognised that men can become depressed both during and following the pregnancy. This chapter explores the effect this may have on relationship issues and asks how can the father emotionally support the mother if he is unable to help himself?

It may be argued that the stereotyping of modern fatherhood often lies between two opposing poles. On one side is the modern concept of the androgynous male who has both masculine and feminine attributes, whilst on the other side is the passive aggressive male, maintaining the authoritarian, absent father stereotype. The reality is probably a combination of the two.

The androgynous male is sometimes portrayed as the popular media stereotype of being a bumbling dad, rather like the father character in the popular television programme, 'The Simpsons'. He embraces and has changed his attitude with the modern expectations of both father involvement and father as the provider. He is supportive to the mother and understands her needs and expectations. He engages with his infant and is often responsible for most of the childcare, giving up his job to look after his infant as his partner is probably a higher wage earner. He has the propensity to seek out any information on child care and enjoys devouring and learning as much as he can. He is not afraid to seek help and will search for appropriate resources, using social medial and websites.

The passive aggressive male may subscribe to the societal gender role whereby the mother is responsible for child rearing, and he has a tendency to an anti-feminine attitude. He may be viewed as being self-reliant, which has been encouraged by his own upbringing and he does not wish to appear feeble. Traditionally he condemns beneficial health-seeking behaviours as an unnecessary pursuit. There is a tendency to avoid seeking help for anything, particularly stress and anxiety, and he prefers to self-manage his condition. Often, he will self-medicate with alcohol and/or drugs as a release from his anxiety or morose condition. For the most part, even if feeling anxious or depressed, he may appear expressionless as the preference is to keep his emotions under control and not to display any signs of weakness. If there is any hint of sympathy or help, this may be met with derision. In order to preserve his 'sanity' he may resort to irritation or aggressive behaviour (Addis & Mahalik 2003).

Status and achievement are important, he does not give in, and will continue to try to manage his life and attempt to achieve whatever is needed within the workplace or at home. The mere sight of a pack of anti-depressants can lead him to re-evaluate his life and reinforces the idea that society is desperate to diagnose a mental condition, rather than encourage men to 'get a grip'. As part of his independence, he will view his situation as a 'catch all' solution for everyday living because he is concerned with the problem of stigma, which he may have experienced in the past.

The reality is a blurring of the roles whereby a combination of both stereotypes is more likely. The father's attitude could be designed by own upbringing, which has encouraged self-reliance. However, this may not always be achievable, and he desperately aspires to be a part of the modern day thinking about behaviours and tries to express his feelings. Although he may be reticent to endorse health-seeking behaviours, he can see the merit in them. He may prefer to keep his emotions in control, and although this may be his preference, he realises that he cannot continue to manage alone with these feelings. He might get irritated if there is any hint of sympathy or help as this may be the first reaction of any man, because it contradicts his own thoughts on how he thinks he should behave. If there is a tendency towards an anti-feminine attitude with 'No girly nonsense, don't appear weak', he secretly concedes that help is really needed. Status and achievement are important, so he will not give in. He will continue to try to manage his life and attempt to achieve whatever is needed in the workplace or at home. However, he may not be able to be as successful as he would like to be because his mood state dictates how he will feel.

He may tend to avoid seeking help and prefer to self-manage the condition (Addis & Mahalik 2003). Often, he will self-medicate; however, once he has re-evaluated it, he may conclude that medication is, in fact, necessary. This can be true of both 'stereotypes' as they may try to self-manage in the first instance. Often, he subscribes to the societal gender role whereby the mother is responsible for child rearing, but recognises he has a part to play, but is not convinced. However, he is prepared to find out more about how to engage with his infant. He is concerned with the problem of stigmatism, and may have experienced this in the past. This will make him more cautious but may also encourage him to learn more about it. He may feel that society is desperate to diagnose rather than encourage men to get a grip. As health services currently stand, that may not be too far from the truth.

Stigma

As the research and studies become more familiar with the process and impact of paternal mental illness on family life, there is an interesting duality. There is no doubt that lifestyle is distinctly impaired because of the changes in mood and function. There is still, however, the problem of stigma and discrimination which can interfere with the father's recovery and social reintegration.

Examining the difference in the attitude of gender stereotypes; stereotypical women are supposed to be kind hearted, caring and emotionally dependent, whilst men are expected to be stoic, decisive, determined, focussed and independent. Weakness is not an option. Should a man violate these expectations and the 'social norms', they will be penalised both socially and economically (Rudman et al. 2012).

The stigma attached to mental illness is a multifaceted process which is associated with serious consequences for the father. The stigmatisation of moderate mental illness does appear to have diminished somewhat over the years, but in cases of the more severe illnesses there is a tendency for stigma to intensify. Reports in the media will sensationalise the actions of the 'mentally ill' criminal. This does not incur a sympathetic approach and understanding from public opinion. It encourages harsh attitudes and calls for the man to be incarcerated and severely punished for his demeanours. A report by the National Audit Commission (2017) stated: *Government does not know how many people in prison have a mental illness, how much it is spending on mental health in prisons or whether it is achieving its objectives. It is therefore hard to see how Government can be achieving value for money in its efforts to improve the mental health and wellbeing of prisoners. In 2016 there were 40,161 incidents of self-harm in prisons and 120 self-inflicted deaths.*

Evidence suggests that men are more likely to suffer from stigma because of their mental illness, which might explain their reluctance to seek treatment (Johnson et al. 2012). There is often an emphasis on labelling, to include the stereotypical attitude, that as he is mentally ill, he must be dangerous, and as a result he is a threat, not only to society, but to himself, his family and particularly his vulnerable infant. His precarious mental state renders him a social outcast and although not always a conscious decision by his fellow mates, he may be aware of their social distancing and avoidance. There is also the preconception that the father must take responsibility for his mental state and his peers may construe this as his weakness. He may face negative emotional reactions which may include angry, sometimes violent interactions from those who fail to understand his motivations. For those who are uncomfortable with the father's behaviour, they may prefer not to interact with him because of their fear or anticipation of the harm he may do to them, even if that is not, and has never been, obvious.

The mentally ill father who fails to perform his paternal duties because of his mood disorders can be penalised with decreased life opportunities, particularly in the work place and loss of independent functioning (Hinshaw & Stier 2008). It is known that the consequences of mental illness stigma can outweigh the impairments associated with psychological disorders themselves (Hinshaw 2007). As a result, he may experience a loss of status, not only within his social circles but within his employment opportunities (Gaebel et al. 2002).

There is much criticism of the 'snowflake generation' who do not possess the 'backbone' or 'stiff upper lip' attitude in adverse situations. They are perceived as weak and vulnerable. Some blame the resilience of former generations which stops the younger age groups from having the liberty to emotionally express themselves. Previously the 'keep calm and carry on' phrase was synonymous with just getting on with it and not getting anxious or complaining. Others may argue that the need to constantly discuss emotions and feelings is the demonization of masculinity and the general oppression of men.

Some of this has been attributed to social media where the crossover of listening to depressed and anxious people sharing innermost emotions on video, can lower the viewer's emotions. This is further exacerbated by the media platforms of Twitter and Instagram now being baited for inciting hatred and animosity by indiscriminate users. Insensitive comments have influenced the father's negative emotions and in some extreme cases this has led to suicidal ideation and in some cases suicide.

There is evidence to suggest that the father who is mentally unwell is less likely to receive high quality or intensive physical health care. Sometimes medical staff fail to diagnose a physical illness because the signs and symptoms may be attributed to the mental illness. This can lead to underdiagnosis and consequently a lack of the correct treatment for his physical condition (Thornicroft et al. 2007).

Studies have found that a depressed masculine stereotype male, suffering from depression, who sought help, experienced less stigma than an identical type male who chose not to seek any help (Moss-Racusin & Miller 2016, Singley & Edwards 2015). This supports the idea that seeking support helps to reduce stigma as it emphasises the fact that that even the most macho of men can suffer from mental illness and are not afraid to access the help they need. One study found that this attitude gained the respect of others, in comparison with those men who chose not to seek help. This information should encourage men to be more forthright and take responsibility about how they feel (Moss-Racusin & Miller 2016).

As more people discuss their experiences of 'mental issues', currently there is a tendency to commend them for sharing their experiences, which have happened often years following an event, with the general public, inferring that they are 'brave' and 'courageous'. There are testimonials and declarations from the rich and famous, and when their journey is shared with the media, the accompanying mellow music and long lingering shots, portray a man who has struggled with adversity and successfully reached the other side. But what of the man who is not courageous or does not feel he can share his story, or his present symptoms? Does that translate as if you are not, or don't feel brave, then you are unable to admit to your mental illness? What message is that conveying to men?

The subject has begun the discussion with, as this book demonstrates, fathers willing to share their story and discuss their journey. It is hoped this will help men to recognise their own disorder or illness and to make the close family and wider community aware of their plight. It has previously been said that being able to find the key in the perinatal period may unlock the mysteries of mental health and illness.

Story of a father and stigma

Rob, was brought up solely by up by his father as his mother was an alcoholic and had left the home when Rob was a baby. His father was a strict disciplinarian, who showed little emotion. Rob's father was a steel worker, and was away from the home for long hours. He despised any signs of weakness and was adamant that his son would be strong and 'man up' to any adversity. This phrase echoed in Rob's ears throughout his childhood. Despite his father's elevated expectations, Rob could never aspire to his father's dreams. Rob loved his father and all he wanted was for his father to be proud of him.

Then during his teenage years, Rob suffered from a bout of depression, but was afraid to admit it in case he was labelled 'mental' or 'mad'. At the age of 47 years, Rob became the father of twins. His depression reoccurred shortly after they were born.

Rob said: I just couldn't speak to my dad or anyone else about how I felt as I was afraid I would totally disgrace my family. I was weak and not a good father to the twins. I have thought I would be better off going abroad in the middle of the night, away from it all and leaving my family, but then I think how bad I felt when my mother was not around for me when I was growing up. I feel I can't get help in case it is recorded on my medical records and I will never get another job and will lose my friends. I can't handle the word depression ever being talked about. I know someone will hear it and I would be devastated if one of the other workers found out about it. Sometimes I don't want to be on this planet anymore, but I will never leave my twins and am hoping it will work out. I just feel I would be discriminated against if I tell anyone else in my community.

The impact on the mother

Whilst in previous generations the role of the mother was to nurture her infant, the father's influence was meant to have a profound effect on the moral and spiritual growth of the child. He provided, in an authoritarian manner, the instructions on the disciplining of the children and would often mete out the sometimes harsh punishments if they disgraced or failed to obey him (Pleck 1997). As with the saying *'spare the rod and spoil the child'* (Proverbs 13:24), fathers believed that children's character would be ruined by over affection. Over forty years ago the societal expectations of the role of childcare between the parents was identified as the cornerstone of normal life, together with the importance of accepting childbirth as a natural event.

Since the 1980s society has acknowledged the advent of the working mother. Although, in the past, some women were responsible for earning a wage outside of the home, the number of mothers who are expected to work, has increased significantly. This has its consequences and it would appear that some women cannot cope with the undue stresses and expectations of today's society.

The patriarchal family slowly diminished, though the timing is indefinite. It is thought that the industrial revolution had a significant impact on the parenting roles because fathers went to work whilst mothers remained at home. It is suspected, however, that many an adult can remember being threatened with *'wait til your father comes home'* for the probability of a beating if they misbehaved. Gradually fathers were expected to chastise less, be more of a teacher of morality, and instil a sense of discipline into the household.

It was during the latter part of the 20th century that saw the demise of the extended family in which the third generation was cared for by the first. The economic pressures required a second income to afford mortgages and other necessities. Women were, from a functional perspective, constrained by common beliefs, accepted that they should stay at home to care for the child, whilst on the other hand they felt obliged to agree with modern day feminist thinking regarding their 'rights' to freedom and the need to accept the triple role of wife, mother and worker. Women redefined their role in society and as a result there were gains and losses, which inevitably affected the childcare responsibilities and the partnership between mothers and fathers. Previously, the father, as a provider for the family, was now subsumed by a joint income with contributions from the mother's employment. The man's status as head of the household and ultimate disciplinarian was waning.

There is evidence to suggest that in order to work, mothers experience significant stress from the tensions arising from straddling the separate spheres of home and work. A recent study found a nearly 40% increase in the stress levels of working mothers, particularly if they have two children and are working full-time (Chandola et al. 2019). Attempts to dilute and devolve their responsibility for the home sphere, as in the case of childcare facilities, have sometimes proved to be expensive and difficult.

With the new forms of social organisation in which all women are expected to work to maintain standards of living and ideologies of equality, they have sought to build a meaningful life for themselves outside of the home. Mothers acknowledged, they had little choice about working because their financial situation dictated that their income was of prime importance to the family. However, working outside of the family home isolates mothers from the domestic environment. In many cases women were unfamiliar with their female counterparts in the community and that they were placed in the unenviable position of being forced to rely on support outside of their normal social circles. Previous support systems appear to have deteriorated, as statistics show that 4.7 million of the workforces have dependent children and the majority of the workforce, in the older age bracket, comprises women. As a result, some women appear to have more commitment to the workplace than the home (Parker 2015).

It is probable that mothers in a previous era would have felt the same pressures and stresses had they shared the same lifestyles of today's mothers. However, the terms of their pregnancy may have differed significantly. There was more emphasis on rest and relaxation to counteract the effects of stress, something that is probably an anathema to the working woman. Unwittingly, society was recognising the dilatory effect of stress and high anxiety, not only on the woman's wellbeing, but that of her unborn infant. In recent years, science has since been uncovering the reality of stress in pregnancy.

The science of epigenetics and neuroscience has revealed some fascinating facts. This is concerned with the familiarity with DNA and inheritance. The influence of environmental factors can affect the DNA and subsequently the development of the foetus. The DNA is instructed about how we will develop and function and also how we are going to develop. Epigenetics changes how it is read and when this is read. The double helix structure of the DNA is familiar, coiled around which are proteins known as istones. The spacing between the istones determines how and if it can be read; it is easier to read with good spacing rather than them being bunched up. The addition of new chemical groups determines whether the actual gene is turned on or off, and when it is turned on, then by how much. In studies with mice, it was found that good nutrition had a more positive effect on the structure. We now know that the structure of the foetus's brain can be altered by the environment within the uterus and this in turn can be affected by the mother's chemistry (Glover et al. 2010, Coussons-Read 2013, Thomason et al. 2017).

During pregnancy, mothers who are subjected to excessive stress means this can adversely affect the development of the foetus. Cortisol, the hormone produced when stress occurs, is particularly important for mediating the effects of the mother's stress, and the placenta acts as a barrier to limit the amount of cortisol the foetus is exposed to, as it is able to filter what passes from the mother to the foetus. The emotional state of the mother, however, can change this filtering capacity. Therefore, the more stress the mother is subjected to, the more of the hormone cortisol is able to pass through, and in turn, can alter the development of the foetal brain (Glover et al. 2010).

For the more exacting science, the cortisol is broken down by an enzyme called11β-HSD2. The enzyme 11-β hydroxysteroid dehydrogenase type 2 (11-βHSD2) converts active cortisol to inactive cortisone. However, increased maternal stress has been shown to reduce placental 11-βHSD2 expression and increase foetal cortisol exposure. Evidence has shown new brain cells are formed well into adulthood, but that during foetal brain construction, it experiences the greatest growth just before birth. One study found a direct association between the gestational age of the foetus and the anxiety which was reported during the third trimester of the pregnancy, resulting in the premature birth of the infant (Langhoff-Roos et al. 2006).

Reflecting on what was known about the effects of stress on the unborn infant, it is then hardly surprising that our pregnant ancestors were given advice by the old wives, whose tales spoke of the importance of avoiding worry, fear or anger as it would influence mother's blood, responsible for the infant's food supply. In some instances, they spoke of the infant suffering an unsightly mark or deformity because the mother suffered shock after she witnessed a horrible sight. The idea was to ensure the mother was prevented from being subjected to any distress. The old wives' tales cautioned the mother to be calm, happy and sweet-tempered, words which hold resonance, as science had discovered the deleterious effect of maternal stress on the foetus. Now it is understood that the hypothalamus/ pituitary/ adrenal axis is responsible for the excessive production of cortisol, which passes through to the foetus. It is also known from studies that this is linked to anxiety, which can result in hyperactivity and some cases, attention deficits in children. A link with ASD has also been suggested. Therefore, there is the likelihood that a man whose mother was anxious, will be anxious himself.

What this all basically means is that the less stress the mother encounters during pregnancy, the better it is for the developing foetus. This has significant implications for the father as it is in his interest to ensure his child has the best possible start in life. It must also be remembered that it is feasible that the father's own mother might have suffered from antenatal anxiety or depression.

The relationship between the father and the infant begins before birth. An unplanned pregnancy can have effects on the father's attitude towards the birth. What of the father's reaction to the foetus? During the six months before the birth of the infant and six months following it, one study found that the depressed father revealed that he had a less positive attitude towards sexual relations, lower satisfaction in his marital relationship and a less positive attitude towards the baby and the pregnancy (Pinto et al. 2017, Bradley & Slade (2011).

Maternal depression has been identified as the strongest predictor of paternal depression (Goodman 2004, Schumacher et al. 2008). It is associated with conflict within their existing relationship coupled with the reality of having a baby together. Marital conflict as a cause of parental depression was explored by Hanington et al. (2012) and found it partially mediated the relationship between postnatal depression in both the mothers and the fathers and in the outcomes for the child. During the antenatal period, parental depression and marital conflict were both associated with adverse effects which persisted even when the postnatal stresses were taken into account. As the mother seeks support from the father, equally the father seeks support from the mother, but if there is disharmony within the relationship and the mother is depressed, this adds to further friction (Deklyen et al. 2006, Mao et al. 2011). Studies have drawn attention to links between the occurrence and severity of postnatal depression and the amount and quality of support that is provided by husbands and by relatives (O'Hara, 1986).

Findings have outlined the gender differences in parenting, which includes the uniqueness of the fathering skills, the interaction between parents and paternal masculinity on the child's outcomes. There is a dominant discourse within society that the father is able to make a uniquely male contribution to the development of the child, particularly the male child. Studies on parenting have primarily focussed on the role of the mother as the caregiver, which has discounted the interdependency and influence of each parent (Ponnet et al. 2013). However, with the advent of the 'new man', it seems that fathers are now more involved in child rearing than they have been in previous generations, and the gap between their own and the mother's participation, is shrinking (Amato et al. 2009).

Over the past forty years the characteristics of fathers have been cited as risk factors for the mother's mental health and the development of the infant. Where there have been studies involving both parents, the onus has been on the health of the mother with very few studies demonstrating the impact of the father's mental health on the mother.

Domestic violence and abuse

Evolutionary theory questions the consequential differential reproduction, explaining that changes can occur only if certain genotypes have a reproductive advantage over others. Evolution is not represented by the survival of the fittest but by the perpetuation of genes. Fitness can be defined only in terms of reproductive success. Evolution has been described as an unconscious existential game, where the objective is to maximise one's genetic representation in subsequent generations.

Burch et al. (2004) argue that paternal uncertainty is one point of departure for applying evolutionary theory to instances of spousal abuse or domestic violence. Domestic abuse is defined as an act of aggression that can be committed by a partner or family member. The abuse can be viewed from an emotional, physical, sexual or financial perspective. All forms of domestic abuse have existed within different cultures for thousands of years. When examining the skulls of mummies, over 3000 years ago, a higher incidence of fractures was found in those of women, compared with men, presumably they were caused as a result of domestic abuse.

Domestic violence is often associated with non-egalitarian decision making (Hampton 1999). It is less visible in equal relationships, which appears to have lower rates of violence, whereas the highest rates are found in affiliations where the male is the dominant partner. This type of relationship is where the male uses all types of abuse to retain and maintain power. Where the male is not dominant, however, they may resort to violence in response to their perceived powerlessness. One study by Devries et al. (2010) of violence during the antenatal period, found that the prevalence for domestic abuse was relatively constant within the fifteen–thirty-five years age group, with a slight decline in the rates after thirty-five years of age. A finding was that intimate partner violence was more common than some of the antenatal health conditions, which are routinely screened for in antenatal care. As she is physically vulnerable, society condemns any harm or abuse of the pregnant woman, yet the occurrence of domestic violence by the male partner appears to escalate during this period. Studies have shown that sexual jealousy also intensified and created the paranoia that the male may not be the father of the child. This is particularly striking, as often the woman in an abusive relationship may believe that her partner will be more sympathetic and less likely to abuse her during her pregnancy (Burch et al. 2004).

It is known that domestic violence is a contributor to postnatal depression, and by that very fact, that it must contribute towards antenatal stress. Studies have shown that domestic violence in the perinatal period is associated with adverse obstetric outcomes, but the evidence is limited on its association with perinatal mental disorders (Romito et al. 2009, Dennis & Vigod 2013, Howard et al. 2013). In one study by Howard et al. (2013) it was established that there was consistent evidence of a high prevalence, with increased odds, of mothers who had experienced domestic violence among those women who experienced anxiety and post-traumatic stress disorder during the perinatal period.

Other studies noted that mothers who suffered with depression during the perinatal period were found to be three times more likely to have been the victims of domestic violence and five times more likely to have experienced violence whilst pregnant. Statistics show that from 2006–2008, 12% of women who died had features of domestic abuse. Prior to their death, others had proactively self-reported domestic abuse to a healthcare professional either before or during their pregnancy (Dennis & Vigod 2013, Howard et al. 2013).

Women as perpetrators of domestic abuse

What is not commonly discussed is that the same tactics used by men against women are also used by women against men. However, there appears to be the little support for male victim of domestic abuse. For example, in England and Wales there are 7,500 spaces in refuges for women; in contrast there are just twenty-three spaces in refuges and eighty-three maximum spaces in safe houses for male partners, around 0.8% of the total (ManKind Initiative 2018). In Scotland and Northern Ireland there are no refuges or safe houses for male victims. It has been quoted that 40% of the victims of domestic abuse are men. Support services, however, are almost non-existent and charitable organisations support this view. Research has shown that men, as either the perpetrator or victims of domestic violence and abuse, present with symptoms of anxiety and depression (Randle and Graham 2011, Hester et al. 2014).

Women often admit they can be equally aggressive in their relationships as men. Some of the literature refers to women who admit to being the sole perpetrator and were as likely as men to be the aggressor (Straus 2005). This is a contentious subject as it is often believed that women use violence as a means of self-defence or because they have an opportunity to be violent towards an abusive partner. These include physical, emotional and verbal threats and the fear, intimidation and shame that is felt as a victim of abuse. Self-defence is often used as a reason for the violent episodes. In this situation the woman is forced to use as much strength as is necessary to defend herself against her aggressor. She may have been oppressed for a considerable time and uses violence to resist further domination.

There are women who use brutality as a powerful tool to control their partner. It has also been found that women initiate and carry out physical assaults on their partners as often as men (Straus 1999, 2005). It is assumed that violence perpetrated by women is relatively harmless with a lower probability of any physical injury. It is, however, more likely to exacerbate a violent situation and cause the man to retaliate, but with a more severe reaction. This is, however, not always the case as women are known to use weapons, to include knives, household objects and boiling water against men. However, because of social taboos, men tend to defend themselves and accept the violence, rather than react. It has been found that these assaults account for up to 40% of injuries. There is still reticence to accept female violence, and men are often faced with bias towards the female, as he must be the perpetrator and the aggressor.

Same sex intimate abuse

It has been argued that men who feel powerless, probably attempt to bolster their fragile sense of masculinity by abusing women in order to maintain their male dominance. Therefore, it is frequently viewed as a gender issue, which occurs between men and women. However, this opinion is contradicted when intimate partner violence occurs between same genders and suggests that power is not the key.

The disparities in the physical size and strength do not seem as important as the ability to control and dominate the relationship (Rohrbaugh 2006). The types of abuse are similar to cross gender relationships with the exception that threats can be used to expose the partner to friends and family, which brings its own challenges and fears, particularly if not everyone is aware of their sexual orientation (Jeffries & Kay 2010, Rolle et al. 2018).

The stigma attached to intimate partner violence is even greater as little has been studied on the subject in order to understand the complexities of the relationship and the several obstacles, including discrimination and shame, which prevent men from getting help (O'Neal & Parry 2015). Even society has not yet made sufficient provision for the protective housing and shelters for gay men and women, whilst the legal system is only beginning to understand the convolutions of intimate partner violence.

The male victim will remain invisible if parity is not evident. Support is not in place for men and societal views and ignorance mean that men are reluctant to look for help and support. This in turn suggests that female perpetuated domestic abuse is not common or widespread which shrouds this epidemic in secrecy, and it appears as if there is no pressure for change.

Story of father and domestic abuse

John was brought up in a violent atmosphere. His father used to hit his mother and she often retaliated by hitting him with the nearest object she could find. John often found himself at the centre of the rows and was often caught up in the anger. John was hit several times by his father and often went to school with bruises. He explained them away by saying he had fallen off his bike or from a tree. He was soon influenced by some delinquent youngsters in his school which led to poor performance in his work. John felt he had no option but to leave the home at the age of sixteen years. He had always loved sport and wanted to become a professional footballer. However, there was a local

Army recruitment drive, and when he was accepted, John saw this as his opportunity to leave home.

John has been in several relationships but they all ended because of his black moods, although he was only violent in one of them, he abhorred any sense of physical abuse. When John met his wife, he promised himself he would never have any cause to hit her. When his son was born it was a traumatic time for him and his wife. His son was poorly following the birth. A few weeks later John was involved in a car accident where he sustained injuries. Although John made a good recovery, he had great difficulty walking. This ended his army career; however, he managed to find a job locally, but it was not what he really wanted.

As time progressed, his wife became disillusioned with their marriage. John started drinking heavily, became hostile and verbally abusive. On one occasion his wife shouted so loudly and aggressively that it stirred memories of his father's behaviour towards him. John reacted and slapped his wife on the face. The instant it occurred John regretted his actions. However, the rows continued and John's recourse was to hit out at his wife, who refused to tolerate her husband's behaviour and their relationship deteriorated rapidly, forcing John and his wife to separate. John was not allowed access to his son and over time any contact reduced significantly.

Relating his experiences, John admitted he regretted his actions but felt a violence over which he had no control. He recognised the reasons for the demise of his marriage and on reflection, he acknowledged that the violence he experienced during his childhood had left a lasting impression. He hated what these life events had done to him and felt that if his mental pain had been recognised at the time then he might have had the support and develop the life skills to help him manage his life. John believed that if he had that this early prevention and support, who knows, he may have been the kind of father to his child that he had always dreamt of being.

Story of a father and domestic abuse 2

When Clive met his wife Janet, they appeared the ideal couple. They enjoyed the same hobbies and loved travelling. Two years after their wedding, their daughter was born. However, Janet suffered from postnatal depression and found it difficult to bond with her daughter. Clive found he was responsible for most of the child care and looking after the housework. He was often exhausted and resented his morose wife lying on the sofa, gazing at the television. Clive tried hard to understand how Janet must be feeling, but he was also aware of how much he was expected to do. It never seemed enough.

Even though Janet had little time for cleaning, she was hypercritical of Clive's attempts. She 'nagged' him persistently about his inability to clean thoroughly or feed his daughter, and this escalated into shouting and screaming. Clive had always been a kind, quiet man and was hurt by the vicious accusations. He suggested his wife calm down, but this was met with derision. Whatever methods Clive used, Janet seemed to become more aggressive, until on one occasion she lifted up a boiling pan of water and threw it at Clive. The water caught his hand and badly burnt his fingers. At the hospital Clive said it was his own fault and returned home to Janet. Clive said he is still with Janet as he is frightened to leave his daughter with her. He hopes one day, Janet will stop being so antagonistic.

Single fathers

Single fathers, in particular, are subject to the similar risk factors for mental health disorders and illness, as those encountered by mothers. As they seem to be in the minority, there is more emphasis on their isolation from groups of other men, particularly as their peers are probably in work. Their social networks and groups are sparse as they are unable to commit time to these pursuits. Some will trust social media to support them through their adversity, but for others it will be a blight on their fathering. They are able to view other fathers' ability to provide material goods and holidays for their infants, whilst their reliance on universal credit prevents them from doing so. This can deepen their own emotions and exacerbate any feelings of failure.

Same sex parenting

One of the many challenges to the assumptions of the ideal, normal family is the increase in the number of same sex families. This has not been without controversy, but is rapidly becoming accepted. However, in the past, gay men as parents have been subjected to discrimination and stigmatisation, which can create anxiety, depression and put a strain on the relationship. There is, however, current evidence which suggests that gay men are competent parents in spite of the challenges they face, and it is the discrimination from the public towards their children that is more harmful than their actual parenting (Parke 2013, Oberklaid 2017).

Whereas it was difficult in the past for same sex couples to adopt children, this has now been relaxed and it tends to be the older males who choose this route. As it is now socially acceptable, and with assisted reproductive technologies, which include egg donor artificial insemination and surrogacy, it is now possible for a same sex couple to become parents. However, there are financial implications and not every couple will be in a position to be able to afford the treatments. Parenting arrangements may also have a more practical route, whereby a woman is contracted to become pregnant for the couple. Sometimes this results in co-parenting with the biological mother and the same sex parents. There are emerging websites which are specifically designed to help same sex couples.

The association between the quality of same sex relationships and depressive symptoms is quite robust and is associated with fewer depressive symptoms. However, where there was greater interdependence, there were stronger concurrent links between depression and the quality of the relationship. One study did not find any gender difference in the association between relationship quality and depressive symptoms. This suggests that stable and happy same sex relationships can promote psychological wellbeing (Whitton & Kuryluk 2014).

The implications on the development of children have been well documented. Despite initial reticence to accept an infant can be raised by a same sex couple, studies have shown that children are not harmed but have normal social, cognitive and emotional development. One study found that children in same sex parent families were significantly less stereotyped in their play than children found in heterosexual families, though this was more marked in lesbian mother families than gay father families. Although gay fathers were stricter and set more limits on their children, they also provided greater reasoning for their decisions (Parke 2013).

Story of a father in a same sex relationship

Stewart in a same sex relationship was struggling after six months following the adoption of his baby boy. Unknown to him, his depression got worse after isolating himself and giving up work, whilst his partner became the breadwinner of the family. Stewart was used to a good social life and but was now feeling tired and stressed. He was unaware of any other parents in a similar situation or parenting classes, and went to the doctor, and was diagnosed with severe depression. After talking with other professionals, it was soon known that he wasn't enjoying parenting and was struggling to bond with his baby boy. He looked back on his previous life and recognised how enjoyable it was. Stewart's relationship was also struggling, but it wasn't until he met a same sex father, who was also diagnosed with postnatal depression that everything made sense. Stewart had not understood what postnatal depression was and was now made aware that if there had not been a baby, he would not have become so depressed.

Impact on the Infant

The impact on the infant appears to begin in the first stages of life. Traditionally, in the neonatal intensive care unit (NICU), health practitioners have paid more attention to the mother than the father. Yet studies have shown that the father wants to be an equal partner and often finds it difficult relating to his new born infant because of his elevated stress levels. The sight of his vulnerable infant can cause both him and his partner feelings of fear anger and guilt; however, it is the mother's emotions which are mostly addressed (Hynan 2005). Recent studies have found there should be more emphasis on the father's inclusion in the care of his infant and his partner by encouraging skin to skin contact and addressing their anxieties too. This early intervention can help the attachment process and significantly reduce the father's anxiety (Schappin et al. 2013, Noergaard et al. 2018).

The legacy of not attending to the father's needs can result in elevated stress levels which impact his employment and domestic life. Recent statistics show that over 91% of fathers who returned to work whilst their infant was in NICU, had difficulty in concentrating, whilst over 20% of fathers had to cease employment to become a full-time carer for their infant (Neonatalmentalhealth).

Some studies found there was an association between the mothers who were anxious when thirty-two weeks pregnant and the long-term behavioural outcomes, and a higher incident of ADHD in the children when they were aged two years to seven years of age (O'Connor et al. 2003, O'Donnell et al. 2014). The studies also suggested that the children were at greater risk of ACEs as teenagers and more likely to develop depression as adults (Stein et al. 2014, Plant et al. 2015). Although the impact of maternal depression on infants has been well documented, until recently there has been little known about the effects of the father's mental health on the infant.

One study looked at the interactions of both parents suffering from anxiety and depression and explored the relationship with their infant at the age of three months. It was found that the mother's response to the infant was less sensitive than if she alone suffered from depression. Anxiety and depression in both parents appear to have an early influence on the quality of the interaction between the mother and the infant (Ramchandani et al. 2005, Lerardi et al. 2018).

Depressed parents have a poorer sense of coherence towards their infant and were more negatively disposed towards their infant and more likely to find the infant's temperament 'difficult', when compared to other infants. Predictably, there was greater impact on the infant's cognitive development because the parents demonstrated less emotional attachment towards the infant which increases the risk of the infant's behavioural and cognitive problems. This may result in the infant having difficulty in responding and also becoming upset when in contact with strangers or in an unfamiliar territory. Also, the infants tended to be fractious and find it difficult to adapt to any new situations.

A comparison was made between the reactions of depressed and non-depressed parents towards their three- to six-month-old infants to determine the difference in the way they interacted. The depressed fathers did not react negatively with their infant but their non-depressed mothers did not demonstrate the best interactive behaviours (Field et al. 1999).

Studies have found that maternal depression is associated with the father's anxiety and their own anxiety traits with the father's anxiety and depression (Paulson et al. 2006, Vismara et al. 2016). These conditions can influence how the mother reacts to the infant and later, to how the infant reacts to the mother. Some men who themselves have an anxiety state and whose partners also suffer from anxiety, may find it difficult to engage with the infant and the mother relationship as they may feel they are intruding on the care and will often withdraw from that type of nurturing. This however, becomes altered when both parents are depressed. They appear to have more stress within the parenting relationship and greater marital dissatisfaction. As one study demonstrated, when parents were interacting face to face with their infants, they tended to show less involvement than the non-depressed parents.

Some depressed fathers felt emotionally detached from their infant and were more likely to admonish their infant, when under a year old, be more critical and were less liable to read to their child (Davis et al. 2011, Bradley & Slade 2011, Kerstis et al. 2013). When talking with infants, the depressed father's speech tended to be focussed on themselves, their negative perceptions and their experiences about their inability to get it right, rather than the experience of the infant. If a crying infant cannot be soothed by him, it is more likely he will blame himself because he was not able to solve or control the situation. In other words, he provides negative reasons for his failure (Sethna et al. 2012, Singley & Edwards 2015).

One study found a difference in the way in which depressed and non-depressed fathers played with their three-month-old infants. The depressed fathers tended to play less excitedly, which included being less capable of making sudden playful noises, producing gestures and movements or funny facial expressions with the infant, and were, overall less gentle and had less active engagement with the infant. However, there was no difference in the way their actual physical play and sensitivity in handling and soothing the infant differed from men who were not depressed. There were occasions, however, when the touching tended to be more vigorous, and on the whole, the occasions when the father did actively engage with the infant were less, compared with the non-depressed fathers. This is in contrast to the earlier findings when fathers' interactions were first studied (Clarke-Stewart 1978, Sethna et al. 2015, Sethna et al. 2018). Whether the fathers played more with their sons than their daughters, remains subject to further research.

The effect of the depressed father seems to be greater than that of any anxious trait the father may exhibit (Aktar et al. 2017). It has also been noted that high depressive symptoms experienced by the father during the postnatal period have been associated with children's emotion regulation problems at three, five and seven years old (Nath et al. 2015). The affected age range has now increased, as a further study found that the father's depression during the postnatal period was associated with their own child's depression at the age of eighteen years and appears to exert its influence on later emotional problems in female children. However, this is thought to be partially explained by the mother being depressed too (Gutierrez-Galve et al. 2019).

Often there is little difference between the way in which both parents talk with their toddler about a crying baby. Both were able to gauge the emotional level of the toddler and knew how to talk about it. However, girls tended towards greater empathic concern for the baby when they were in the presence of their father than they were with the mother. Possible causes for this have suggested that perhaps the girls do not witness the fathers soothing the baby as their mother would have done (McHarg et al. 2019). Parenting interventions on sensitive and responsive care were used with educated mothers.

Educated mothers took part on a parenting intervention course which promoted sensitive and responsive care towards their infant. Although the father was not directly involved with the interventions, it appeared that the mother's participation enhanced the infant's cognitive and socioemotional development whilst the input from the father only influenced the infant's socioemotional development. However, it was found that the input of the father influenced the mother's ability to parent, despite the fact they were the primary carers in the study (Jeong et al. 2019).

The father's overall behaviour is more likely to be dictated by his own interests in the interaction with the infant and not in response or dictated to by the needs of his infant. This suggests the father's depressed mood and his difficulty with social behaviour has an impact on how he interacts with his infant. It could also be explained by the symptoms of depression which include the lack of sleep and low energy levels which would make him less inclined to be playful with the infant. The timings of the father's interactions have also been studied and during the father's rest days, his engagement in play predicted greater attachment to the infant, as compared to the days when he was working (Brown et al. 2018).

One of the foibles of depression is that it has a tendency to become self-absorbing and self-focussed. Often depressed parents ruminate on their own feelings rather than those of their children. This necessitates the need for more research into the family environment. This acts as a pathway for risk transmission from fathers to children. The depressed father is associated with adverse outcomes for his infant. That and conflict within the partnership between the parents is also a risk factor for childhood behavioural problems. Therefore, the quality of support offered to the mother from the father is vital to establish and maintain a healthy relationship and provide a nurturing environment for the infant (Sethna et al. 2015).

Story of a father and his infant

Carl, a 33-year-old single father, was left to bring up his infant son alone after his girlfriend abandoned them both. He didn't think about it at the time, but he refused to ask for any help as he was worried that social services would become involved. He said he was 'really down and lonely'. He could not go out to work as he had no family living close to him and he had to be a full-time father. Finances were tight and Carl deprived himself of necessities in order to provide for his son. He ensured that his son's physical needs were catered for and that he was well clothed and had all the equipment.

On reflection, he recognised that he did not engage with his son as much as he should have done. Carl found he was less tactile and limited playtime to only a few minutes at a time. He got cross when his son would not stop crying and blamed everything and everyone but himself for his son's poor behaviour. Eventually he found it easier to ignore his son's cries and invested in a games console to take his mind off what was happening in the home. Carl said 'I didn't think anything of it at the time, but I was ignoring my son and didn't really want to attend to his needs, which now makes me feel guilty. I am working part time and as a result am a happier father now. My son is eight years old and he seems very happy, but gets angry on times and can't keep still when he is in school or at home'.

Adverse childhood experiences

There is now significant emphasis on adverse childhood experiences (ACEs) and the correlation between this and adult mental health is becoming well established. There are, however, several complex issues which determine how these early experiences can impact later life. This influence is probably more elaborate and multifaceted than has been understood in the past, and that during adulthood, these factors can attribute to poor financial outcomes, lack of social support and impairment in mental health (Jones et al. 2018).

The incidence of adults having at least one ACE is variable and relatively common, whilst some estimates are almost 70% (Wade et al. 2016). The experiences of children who may have lived in a dysfunctional family and have witnessed domestic violence and drug abuse or who have been subjected to physical, sexual and emotional abuse and neglect, are at an increased risk of anxiety and depression. They are more likely to exhibit aggressive behaviour, be prone to taking illicit substances and more at risk of suicidal tendencies (Petchel & Pizzagalli 2011, Nurius et al. 2015).

Although it is accepted that adverse childhood experiences have a significant effect on the mental health outcomes for the child in adulthood, there are only a few studies which have looked at the complexities of the ways in which this can manifest (Jones et al. 2018). Those studies which have explored the outcomes for children found that those with four or more determinable ACEs are twice as likely to have a poor diet, three times more likely to smoke, five more time likely to engaged in sex under the age of sixteen years and boys are six times more likely to accidently cause a pregnancy (Bellis et al. 2014, 2017).

There is also evidence to suggest that those with four ACEs are twice as likely to binge drink, seven times more likely to be involved in recent violence, eleven times more likely to have been incarcerated and more likely to have used illicit substances such as heroin or crack cocaine (Bellis et al. 2014). In whatever sphere of lifestyles that are studied particularly in relation to related to health issues, there appears to be an increase in the number of hospital attendances, visits to the general practitioner and dentist (Ford et al. 2016).

Being brought up in a household that has a low income, sometimes manifesting as poverty, has its own challenges for the child, because poverty can predict increased physiological problems in adulthood, irrespective of any concurrent risks that the adult may be exposed to. Structural constraints may cause the family to struggle to provide adequate nutrition and choose negative health behaviours, ultimately leading to diminished emotional resources. This suggests that some of the pathways from adulthood to that of mental health may carry biological as well as socio-structural effects from the early hardships of abuse, family dysfunction and poverty (Evans & Kim 2012). This adversity can impact studying and lead to lower educational attainment, resulting in lower socioeconomic achievement in adulthood. It can also affect the breadth and quality of existing and future social networks (Font & Maguire-Jack 2016).

It is understood that if the mother experiences stress during her pregnancy this can have an adverse effect on her unborn child; it is also known that stress in childhood is a risk factor for subsequent mental health problems in later life. Continuous exposure to such situations can cause stress damage to physiological resources (Wickrama et al. 2014). Prolonged exposure to stress increases the stress hormone levels and the hypothalamic, pituitary adrenal (HPA) axis dysregulation. Adults who have been exposed to abuse during their childhood have had increased levels of inflammation and HPA activation.

This overload of stress results in what is now termed 'toxic stress'. This is damaging and causes problems in brain development in the child exposed to it. The constant stress reduces the neural connections in the brain, which has consequences for development. Whilst one study suggested that the greater the duration of childhood spent in poverty, with all the stresses that it incurs, the greater the exposure to cumulative risk (Evans & Kim 2012, 2013). Therefore, children who live where there is significant deprivation are more likely to be at risk of an ACE.

When under stress the body's natural reaction is to produce cortisol in order to prepare for flight or fight. The heart rate increases and so does the blood pressure to allow the body to react quickly to any impending danger. This is a positive stress response and is normal. An example of which is when the infant is introduced to the new puppy, he is frightened by the unfamiliarity of the animal. Most children can learn how to cope with the perceived danger or adversity with the help of their parent or an adult who will assure and or reassure them that they will protect them, or negate the harmful fear or terror they are experiencing.

The second degree of stress is called a tolerable stress response and is that felt by a child when they are subjected to a situation that even the adult cannot make better, an example of which would be a bereavement or injury. With assurance from an adult, which acts as a buffer from the emotional pain, the time of stressfulness is limited and eventually the child is able to adapt to the situation, allowing the brain and other functions to recover.

If, however, that support is missing, and the fear or stress is not minimised, as for example in the case of abuse, and remains a constant, then this can have repercussions, having a significant effect on brain and other bodily systems. Chronic exposure to stress is termed a toxic stress response, and this can ultimately have an effect throughout the child's life, not only in terms of physical damage but it affects their mental health too. This remains a constant throughout their life, increasing the risk of stress related diseases and cognitive impairment (Hughes et al. 2016).

One study on the impact on mothers found that their ACEs were significantly associated with the children's development. It is now understood that more attention should be paid to the process of how stress is accumulated across the lifespan. Growing up in these negative environments is likely to influence the selection of similar social environments in adulthood and may result in negative pathways already mentioned. The important point is that this proliferation of stress operates through the biosocial pathways and increases the HPA activity, which results in neurobiological dysregulation (Lu et al. 2008, Juster et al. 2010). Therefore, tackling intergenerational adversity amongst young parents may help to promote child development (Sun et al. 2017).

Avid campaigning and tales of mental adversity and the impact this has had on the young, have coerced some governments into putting greater consideration into mental health. There remains, however, insufficient investment into mental health and illness suggesting that either treating a mental illness is still not a priority or is unworkable in the light of more pressing physical problems. Some are content with 'let's put a sticking plaster on it' adage without addressing the real issues. Currently the statistics are not encouraging and suggest that 20% of adolescents may experience a mental health problem in any given year. It has been estimated that half of those problems will be established by the time they are aged fourteen, and this rises to three quarters by the age of twenty-four. What is worrying is that 10% of children aged from five–sixteen years have been diagnosed with a mental disorder, yet over three quarters of those have not had an early intervention (WHO 2003, DOH 2005).

Suicide rates amongst adolescents appear to have increased more than four times the national rate and has risen by 105% in the past five years. These worrying statistics reveal that it is a fact that children have to be suicidal before they are referred to the NHS, and it is often an eighteen-month waiting time before they can see a specialist.

Recognising the impact on the mother and the scarcity of studies on the father's adverse childhood events, it is pertinent to consider screening for ACEs. Once established that there have been traumatic events which could influence the mental health of the parents, appropriate help and support when the infant arrives should be considered. If the screening is neglected in the antenatal period, then consideration should be given during the postnatal period to mitigate any further intergenerational adversity (Hillis et al. 2010).

If the mental health effects of ACEs are absolute or if they might be more adjustable by exposure to healthier social contexts across children's development or whether through specified interventions, then those interventions across several points during the child's lifetime would be beneficial (Turner et al. 2016). Whatever the case, tackling mental health problems at an early age appears to prevent mental health problems at an older age. The next generation should not be failed.

References

Addis ME, Mahalik JR. 2003. Men, masculinity, and the contexts of help seeking. *American Psychologist*, 58, pp. 5–14.

Aktar E, Colonnesi C, de Vente W, Majdandžić M, Bögels SM. 2017. How do parents' depression and anxiety, and infants' negative temperament relate to parent-infant face-to-face interactions? *Development and Psychopathology*, 29, pp. 697–710.

Amato PR, Meyers CE, Emery RE. 2009. Changes in nonresident father–child contact from 1976 to 2002. *Family Relations*, 58(1), pp. 41–53.

Bellis MA, Hughes K, Hardcastle K, Ashton K, Ford K, Quigg Z, Davies A. 2017. The impact of adverse childhood experiences on health service use across the life course using a retrospective cohort study. *Journal of Health Services Research and Policy*, 22(3), pp. 168–177. http://journals.sagepub.com/doi/pdf/10.1177/1355819617706720

Bellis MA, Hughes K, Leckenby N, Perkins C, Lowey H. 2014. National household survey of adverse childhood experiences and their relationship with resilience to health-harming behaviours in England. *BMC Medicine*, 12, p. 72. doi:10.1186/1741-7015-12-72

Bradley R, Slade P. 2011. A review of mental health problems in fathers following the birth of a child. *Journal of Reproductive and Infant Psychology*, 29, pp. 19–42.

Brown GL, Mangelsdorf SC, Shigeto A, Wong MS. 2018. Associations between father involvement and father–child attachment security: Variations based on timing and type of involvement. *Journal of Family Psychology*, 32(8), pp. 1015–1024.

Burch RL, Gordon G, Gallup GG Jr. 2004. Pregnancy as a stimulus for domestic violence. *Journal of Family Violence*, 19(4), pp. 243–247.

Chandola T, Booker CL, Kumari M, Benzeval M. 2019. Are flexible work arrangements associated with lower levels of chronic stress-related biomarkers? A study of 6025 employees in the UK. Household Longitudinal Study. *Sociology*. 53(4), pp. 779–799.

Clarke-Stewart K. 1978. And daddy makes three: The father's impact on mother and young child. *Child Development*, 49(2), pp. 466–478.

Coussons-Read ME. 2013. Effects of prenatal stress on pregnancy and human development: Mechanisms and pathways. *Obstetric Medicine*, 6(2), pp. 52–57.

Davis RN, Davis MM, Freed GL, Clark SJ. 2011. Fathers' depression related to positive and negative parenting behaviors with 1-year-old children. *Pediatrics*, 127(4), pp. 612–618.

Dennis CL, Vigod S. 2013. The relationship between postpartum depression, domestic violence, childhood violence, and substance use: Epidemiologic study of a large community sample. *Violence Against Women*, 19(4), pp. 503–517.

Department of Health DOH & Scottish Exec. 2005. Mental Health of children and young people in Great Britain. https://sp.ukdataservice.ac.uk/doc/5269/mrdoc/pdf/5269technicalreport.pdf, accessed 18 October 2019.

Deklyen M, Brooks-Gunn J, Mclanahan S, Knab J. 2006. The mental health of married, cohabiting, and non-coresident parents with infants. *American Journal of Public Health*, 96(10), pp. 1836–1841.

Devries KM, Kishor S, Johnson H, Stockl H, Baccus LJ, Garcia Moreno C, Watts C. 2010. Intimate partner violence during pregnancy: Analysis of prevalence data from 19 countries. *Reproductive Health Matters*, 18(3), pp. 158–170.

Evans GW, Kim P. 2012. Childhood poverty and young adults' Allostatic load: The mediating role of childhood cumulative risk exposure. *Psychological Science*, 23(9), pp. 979–983.

Evans GW, Kim P. 2013. Childhood poverty, chronic stress, self-regulation, and coping. *Child Development Perspectives*, 7(1), pp. 43–48.

Field TM, Hossain Z, Malphurs J. 1999. Depressed' fathers' interactions with their infants. *Infant Mental Health Journal*, 20(3), pp. 322–332.

Font SA, Maguire-Jack K. 2016. Pathways from childhood abuse and other adversities to adult health risks: The role of adult socioeconomic conditions. *Child Abuse & Neglect*, 51, pp. 390–399.

Ford K, Butler N, Hughes K, Quigg Z, Bellis MA. 2016. Adverse Childhood Experiences (ACEs) in Hertfordshire, Luton and Northamptonshire. https://www.researchgate.net/publication/302589403_Adverse_Childhood_Experiences_ACEs_in_Hertfordshire_Luton_and_Northamptonshire, accessed 19 November 2019.

Gaebel WW, Baumann AA, Witte AM, Zaeske HH. 2002. Public attitudes towards people with mental illness in six German cities: Results of a public survey under special consideration of schizophrenia. *European Archives of Psychiatry and Clinical Neuroscience*, 252(6), pp. 278–287.

Glover V, O'Connor TG, O'Donnell K. 2010. Prenatal stress and the programming of the HPA axis. *Neuroscience and Biobehavioral Reviews*, 35, pp. 17–22.

Goodman JH. 2004. Paternal postpartum depression, its relationship to maternal postpartum depression, and implications for family health. *Journal of Advanced Nursing*, 45(1), pp. 26–35.

Gutierrez-Galve L, Stein A, Hanington L, Heron J, Lewis G, O'Farrelly C, Ramchandani PG. 2019. Association of Maternal and Paternal Depression in the Postnatal Period with Offspring Depression at Age 18 Years. *JAMA Psychiatry*, 76(3), pp. 290–296.

Hampton RL. 1999. *Family Violence Prevention and Treatment*, 2nd ed. New York: Sage Publications.

Hanington L, Heron J, Stein A, Ramchandani P et al. 2012. Parental depression and child outcomes – is marital conflict the missing link? *Child Care Health and Development*, 38(4), pp. 520–529.

Hester M, Ferrari G, Jones SK, Williamson E, Bacchus LJ, Peters TJ, Feder G. 2014. Occurrence and impact of negative behaviour, including domestic violence and abuse, in men attending UK primary care health clinics: A cross-sectional survey. *General practice/Family practice BJM Open access*, 5, p. 5.

Hillis SD, Anda RF, Dube SR, Felitti VJ, Marchbanks PA, Marks JS. 2004. The association between adverse childhood experiences and adolescent pregnancy, long-term psychosocial consequences and fetal death. *Pediatrics*, 113(2), pp. 320–327.

Hillis SD, Anda RF, Dube SR et al. 2010. The protective effect of family strengths in childhood against adolescent pregnancy and its long-term psychosocial consequences. *The Permanente Journal*, 14(3), pp. 18–27.

Hinshaw, SP. 2007. *The Mark of Shame: Stigma of Mental Illness and an Agenda for Change*. New York, NY: Oxford University Press.

Hinshaw SP, Stier A. 2008. Stigma as related to mental disorders. *Clinical Psychology*, 4, pp. 367–393.

Howard L, Oram S, Galley H, Treveillion K, Feder G. 2013. Domestic violence and perinatal mental disorders: A systematic review and meta-analysis. *PLOS*. https://doi.org/10.1371/journal.pmed.1001452

Hughes K, Lowey H, Quigg Z, Bellis MA. 2016. Relationships between adverse childhood experiences and adult mental wellbeing: Results from an English national household survey. *BMC Public Health*, 16, p. 222.

Hynan MT. 2005. Supporting fathers during stressful times in the nursery: An evidence-based review. *Newborn and Infant Nursing Reviews*, 5(2), pp. 87–92.

Jeffries S, Kay M. 2010. Homophobia, heteronormativism and hegemonic masculinity: Male same-sex intimate violence from the perspective of Brisbane service providers. *Psychiatry Psychology and Law*, 17, pp. 412–423.

Jeong J, Obradović J, Rasheed M, McCoy DC, Fink G, Yousafzai AK. 2019. Maternal and paternal stimulation: Mediators of parenting intervention effects on preschoolers' development. *Journal of Applied Developmental Psychology*, 60, pp. 105–118.

Johnson JL, Oliffe JL, Kelly MT, Galdas P, Ogrodniczuk JS. 2012. Men's discourse on help-seeking in the context of depression. *Sociology of Health & Illness*, 35, pp. 346–361.

Jones TM, Nurius P, Song C, Fleming CM. 2018. Modeling life course pathways from adverse childhood experiences to adult mental health. *Child Abuse & Neglect*, 80, pp. 32–40.

Juster RP, McEwen BS, Lupien SJ. 2010. Allostatic load biomarkers of chronic stress and impact on health and cognition. *Neuroscience & Biobehavioral Reviews*, 35(1), pp. 2–16.

Kerstis B, Engstrom G, Elund B, Aarts C. 2013. Association between mothers' and fathers' depressive symptoms, sense of coherence and perception of their child's temperament in early parenthood in Sweden. *Scandinavian Journal of Public Health*, 41(3), pp. 233–239.

Langhoff J, Kesmodel U, Jacobsson B, Rasmussen S, Vogel I. 2006. Spontaneous preterm delivery in primiparous women at low risk in Denmark: Population based study. *British Medical Journal*, 332(5747), pp. 937–939.

Lerardi E, Ferro V, Trovato A, Tambelli R, Crugnloa CR. 2018. Maternal and paternal depression and anxiety: Their relationship with mother-infant interactions at 3 months. *Archives of Women's Mental Health*, 22(4), pp. 527–533.

Lu W, Mueser KT, Rosenberg SD, Jankowski MK. 2008. Correlates of adverse childhood experiences among adults with severe mood disorders. *Psychiatric Services*, 59(9), pp. 1018–1026.

ManKind initiative Charity. 2018. A charity for victims of domestic abuse. www.ManKind.org.uk

Mao Q, Zhu L, Su X. 2011. A comparison of postnatal depression and related factors between Chinese new mothers and fathers. *Journal of Clinical Nursing*, 20(5–6), pp. 645–652.

McHarg G, Fink E, Hughes C. 2019. Crying babies, empathic toddlers, responsive mothers and fathers: Exploring parent-toddler interactions in an empathy paradigm. *Journal of experimental child psychology*, 179, pp. 23–37.

Moss-Racusin CA, Miller HG. 2016. "Taking charge" of stigma: Treatment seeking alleviates mental illness stigma targeting men. *Journal of Applied Social Psychology*. 46(6), pp. 319–335.

Nath S, Russell G, Ford T, Kuyken W, Psychogiou, L. 2015. Postnatal paternal depressive symptoms associated with fathers' subsequent parenting: Findings from the Millennium Cohort Study. *The British Journal of Psychiatry*, 207(6), pp. 558–559.

National Audit office. 2017. *Mental Health in Prisons*, ISBN: 9781786041265 HC: 42, 2017–18.

Noergaard B, Ammentorp J, Garne E, Fenger-Gron J, Kofoed PE, Dowling D, Thibeau S. 2018. Fathers' stress in a neonatal intensive care unit. *Advances in Neonatal Care*, 18(5), pp. 413–422.

Nurius PS, Green SP, Logan-Greene LP, Borja S. 2015. Life course pathways of adverse childhood experiences toward adult psychological well-being: A stress process analysis. *Child Abuse & Neglect*, 45, pp. 143–153.

Oberklaid F. 2017. The kids are OK: It is discrimination, not same-sex parents that harms children. *Medical Journal of Australia*, 207(9), pp. 374–375.

O'Connor TG, Heron J, Golding J, Glover V, ALPAC Study Team. 2003. Maternal antenatal anxiety and behavioural/emotional problems in children: A test of a programming hypothesis. *Journal of Child Psychology and Psychiatry*, 44(7), pp. 1025–1036.

O'Donnell KJ, Glover V, Barker ED, O'Connor TG. 2014. The persisting effect of maternal mood in pregnancy on childhood psychopathology. *Development and Psychopathology*, 26(2), pp. 393–403.

O'Hara MW. 1986. Social support, life events, and depression during pregnancy and the puerperium. *Archives of General Psychiatry*, 43(6), pp. 569–573.

O'Neal EM, Parry MM. 2015. Help-seeking behavior among same-sex intimate partner violence victims: An intersectional argument. *Criminology, Criminal Justice Law and Society*, 16, pp. 51–67.

Parke RD. 2013. *Future Families: Diverse Forms, Rich Possibilities*, 1st ed. USA: John Wiley & Sons, Inc.

Parker K. 2015. Women more than men adjust their careers for family life. FACTANK. https://www.theatlantic.com/politics/archive/2015/10/women-more-often-choose-family-over-work/433029/, accessed 18 October 2019.

Paulson JF, Dauber S, Leiferman JA. 2006. Individual and combined effects of postpartum depression in mothers and fathers on parenting behavior. *Pediatrics*, 118, pp. 659–668.

Petchel P, Pizzagalli DA. 2011. Effects of early life stress on cognitive and affective function: An integrated review of human literature. *Psychopharmacology* , 214, pp. 55–70.

Pinto TM, Samorinha C, Tendais I, Nunes-Costa R, Figueiredo B. 2017. Paternal adjustment and paternal attitudes questionnaire. *Antenatal and Postnatal Portuguese Versions*, 24(6), pp. 820–830.

Plant DT, Pariante CM, Sharp D, Pawlby S. 2015. Maternal depression during pregnancy and offspring depression in adulthood: Role of child maltreatment. *The British Journal of Psychiatry*, 207(3), pp. 213–220.

Pleck JH. 1997. Paternal involvement: Levels, sources, and consequences. In: Lamb ME. (Ed), *The Role of the father in Child Development* (pp. 66–103). Hoboken, NJ: John Wiley & Sons Inc.

Ponnet K, Mortelmans D, Wouters E, Van Leeuwen K, BastaitsInge K, Pasteels I. 2013. Parenting stress and marital relationship as determinants of mothers' and fathers' parenting. *Personal Relationships*, 20(2), pp. 259–276.

Ramchandani P, Stein A, Evans J, O'Connor TG, the ALSPAC study team. 2005. Paternal depression in the postnatal period and child development: A prospective population study, *The Lancet*, 365(9478), pp. 2201–2205.

Randle AA, Graham CA. 2011. A review of the evidence on the effects of intimate partner violence on men. *Psychology of Men and Masculinity*, 12, pp. 97–111.

Rohrbaugh JB. 2006. *Same-Gender Domestic Violence Family Court Review Association of Family and Conciliation Courts*. Oxford: Blackwell Publishing Ltd.

Rolle L, Giardina G, Caldarera AM, Gerinao E, Brustia P. 2018. When intimate partner violence meets same sex couples: A review of same sex intimate partner violence. *Frontiers in Psychology*, 9, p. 1506.

Romito P, Pomicino L, Lucchetta C, Scrimin F, Turan JM. 2009. The relationships between physical violence, verbal abuse and women's psychological distress during the postpartum period. *Journal of Psychosomatic Obstetrics & Gynecology*, 30, pp. 115–121.

Rudman LA, Moss-Racusin CA, Glick P, Phelan JE. 2012. 4 reactions to vanguards: Advances in backlash theory. *Advances in Experimental Social Psychology*, 45, pp. 167–227.

Schappin R, Wijnroks L, Uniken Venema MM, Jongmans MJ. 2013. Rethinking stress in parents of preterm infants: A meta-analysis. *PLOS ONE*, 8(2), p. e54992.

Schumacher M, Zubaran C, WhiteBringing G. 2008. Birth-related paternal depression to the fore. *Women and Birth: Journal of the Australian College of Midwives*. 21(2), pp. 65–70.

Sethna V, Murray L, Edmondson O, Iles J, Ramchandani PG. 2018. Depression and playfulness in fathers and young infants: A matched design comparison study. *Journal of Affective Disorders*, 229, pp. 364–370.

Sethna S, Murray L, Netsi E, Psychogiou L, Ramchandani PG. 2015. Paternal depression in the postnatal period and early father–infant interactions. *Parenting Science and Practice*, 15, pp. 1–8.

Sethna V, Murray L, Ramchandani P. 2012. Depressed fathers' speech to their 3-month-old infants: A study of cognitive and mentalizing features in paternal speech. *Psychological Medicine*, 42(11), pp. 2361–2371.

Singley D, Edwards L. 2015. Men's perinatal mental health in the transition to fatherhood. *Professional Psychology: Research and Practice*, 46(5), pp. 309–316.

Stein A, Pearson RM, Goodman SH, Rapa E, Rahman A, McCallum M, Howard LM, Pariante CM. 2014. Effects of perinatal mental disorders on the fetus and child. *The Lancet*, 384(9956), pp. 1800–1819.

Straus MA. 1999. The controversy over domestic violence by women: A methodological and theoretical and sociology of science analysis. In: Arriaga X, Oskamp S. (Eds), *Violence in Intimate Relationships*. Thousand Oaks, CA: Sage, pp. 17–44.

Straus MA. 2005. Women's violence toward men is a serious social problem. In: Loseke DR, Gelles RJ, Cavanaugh MM. (Eds), *Current Controversies on Family Violence*, 2nd ed. Newbury Park: Sage Publications, pp. 55–77.

Sun J, Patel F, Rose-Jacobs R, Frank DA, Black MM, Chilton M. 2017. Mothers' adverse childhood experiences and their young children's development. *American Journal of Preventive Medicine*, 53(6), pp. 882–891.

Thomason M, Hect JL, van den Heuvel M et al. 2017. High stress in pregnant mothers is associated with reduced global brain efficiency in the fetus. *Biological Psychiatry Supplement*, 81(10), pp. 298–299.

Thornicroft G, Rose D, Kassam A. 2007. Discrimination in health care against people with mental illness. *International Review of Psychology*, 19, pp. 113–122.

Turner R, Thomas C, Brown T. 2016. Childhood adversity and adult health: Evaluating intervening mechanisms. *Social Science & Medicine*, 156, pp. 114–124.

Vismara L, Rollè L, Agostini F et al. 2016. Perinatal parenting stress, anxiety, and depression outcomes in first-time mothers and fathers: A 3- to 6-months' postpartum follow-up study. *Frontiers in Psychology*, 7, p. 938.

Wade R, Cronholm PF, Fein JA, Forke CM, Davis MB, Harkins-Schwarz M, Bair-Merritt MH. 2016. Household and community-level adverse childhood experiences and adult health outcomes in a diverse urban population. *Child Abuse & Neglect*, 52, pp. 135–145.

Whitton SW, Kuryluk AD. 2014. Associations between relationship quality and depressive symptoms in same-sex couples. *Journal of Family Psychology*, 28(4), pp. 571–576.

WHO. 2003. *Caring for Children and Adolescents with Mental Disorders: Setting WHO Directions*. [online] Geneva: World Health Organization.

Wickrama KK, Lee TK, O'Neal CW, Kwon JA. 2014. Stress and resource pathways connecting early socioeconomic adversity to young adults' physical health risk. *Journal of Youth and Adolescence*, 44(5), pp. 1109–1124.

Chapter 3

Exploring the types and manifestation of disorders

Anxiety

Anxiety is an important physical response which is designed to keep the body safe from external harmful stimuli. The 'flight or fight' action motivates the body to act quickly in the face of danger by either avoiding or confronting threatening factors. Short term stress can improve alertness and memory, whereas chronic or severe stress can have harmful affects both physically and mentally.

The neuroscience

The emotions are governed by the limbic system, which is located in the mid brain. Its primary structures include the amygdala, hippocampus, thalamus, hypothalamus, basal ganglia, and cingulate gyrus. The amygdala is the emotion centre of the brain, whilst the hippocampus plays an essential role in the formation of new memories about past experiences. The hypothalamus is found beneath the thalamus and is responsible for releasing hormones. The thalamus is located above the brain stem, between cerebral cortex and the midbrain and is responsible to relay motor and sensory signals to the cerebral cortex. Basal ganglia are a group of neurons and are strongly connected to other areas within the brain. They fine tune the activity within the brain circuits and process information on voluntary body movement, learning, cognition and emotions. The cingulate gyrus is involved in processing and regulating emotions and behaviour (Morgan 2005, Markowitch & Staniloiu 2011). Information is processed and transmitted to the pre-frontal cortex which helps in decision making.

One of the reasons suggested for the symptoms of anxiety is that they are caused by the signalling changes within the limbic system. Brain imaging has revealed that those with anxiety disorders have more activity than normal within the limbic system. The amygdala, in particular, was found to be overly active and larger in size, indicating it may have to process more information than usual and probably accounts for the inability to control the feelings of panic and fear. Although this type of brain imagery is relatively new, it has been found that there are differing activities associated with different disorders. It has been suggested that this may be caused by low levels of the neurotransmitter GABA, which blocks the impulses between the nerve cells in the brain. Therefore, it is even harder to control the feelings of panic and fear.

Anxiety in the father

Disproportionate anxiety, not caused by any external stimuli, is pathological. There are variations in the symptoms for anxiety, with a comprehensive list of the possible signs, but there appears to be no consensus on the definition or threshold for treatments. For most fathers it is difficult for them to determine what is a normal stress response and what is abnormal; therefore, it is problematic for them to determine if they need help or it is something that they should be able to control.

The dominant symptoms of clinically diagnosed anxiety (WHO 2018) are highly variable and sometimes difficult to differentiate. The father may have the continuous feelings of being on edge, waiting for something to happen, but not knowing what. This insecurity may make him react with irritation, frustration or anger. He dismisses the light headedness which causes dizziness and his palpitations, as the need to 'get a grip'. He pays little attention to muscular tension and epigastric pain because of something he must have eaten or some strenuous exercise regime. These symptoms can often be severe and last for several weeks or even months, but may be relieved with alcohol or illicit drugs. The vagueness of some of the symptoms can make it difficult for the father to interpret them as a psychological illness and often, unless he is alerted to the fact by someone who is vigilant about the father's overall behaviour, he will blame outside stimuli and the environment for his condition.

Social phobia

There are several types of anxiety. Social phobia is common. This usually starts in adolescence but the causes are vague. The father may dislike the notion that he is being analysed and assessed by people, particularly within small groups. This engenders his anxious symptoms, and the preference is to avoid social gatherings rather than be subjected to scrutiny of the group. The avoidance may be discreet, by shunning public events, or diffuse, by being selective about with whom and where he socialises. It is often associated with the father having low esteem or having a significant fear of criticism. It is thought the exposure to images and faces produces extra activity in the amygdala. Hence the information is processed through a layer of fear. In some cases, the enormity of the emotions felt may lead to a panic attack.

Panic attacks

Panic attacks are not restricted to a particular situation or set of circumstances (WHO 2018) and are characterised by the sudden onset of breathing problems, persons often finding it difficult to catch their breath, choking sensations, dizziness and feelings of depersonalisation. Palpitations and chest pains are often a feature, and the fear of impending death is not uncommon. Although the father will be able to function fairly normally, his emotions are often in turmoil because of the continuing fear and embarrassment of having a further panic attack in public.

Stress and the foetus

There is significant evidence to suggest that high levels of prolonged stress have implications for the mother and her developing foetus, but there are few studies on the anxiety of the father (Glover 2014). Naturally, as the father has little, biologically, to do with the foetus's development, the impact of his stress presumably does not count. However, it is the impact of the father's stress and anxiety on the mother that can have important influences.

It has been suggested that mothers who have heightened fear about the actual birth process would prefer to have a caesarean section. This fear, if not ameliorated by the father, can result in the mother insisting on the procedure (Rubertsson et al. 2014). It is accepted that breastfeeding can be compromised by maternal anxiety and can have a negative impact on the production and flow of breast milk (Stuebe et al. 2012). Therefore, the father's input to assist the mother with any apprehensions is imperative.

Story of a father with anxiety

Four years ago, Joseph found he was going to be a father. He was there when his girlfriend had a traumatic birth and sadly the baby died in the labour ward. He could remember seeing his girlfriend's and baby daughter's faces, images which haunt him today.

Joseph felt that they did not receive any support or bereavement counselling. The relationship did not last long afterwards. Joseph had lost both his girlfriend and his daughter within the space of weeks. He said that following the events, he had become a totally difference person.

Two years ago, Joseph found love and married, but he felt he wasn't ready to be a dad and worried that the same events would reoccur. He could not confide in his wife, and each time he thought of the events, Joseph became anxious. He found it difficult to relax or to sleep as his mind was always racing. He found himself waking up at night covered in sweat. He put his lack of sleep down to his inability to concentrate. He continually had headaches which he blamed for his stupid mistakes which made him angry.

Inevitably his wife became pregnant, and Joseph found his anxiety increasing substantially. In his head he felt he would lose both of them. He tried to block out his emotions but they were invasive and he could not make them go away.

He was constantly asking his wife how she felt. He would phone her at work and when she was out with friends, but was unaware how anxious he was making his wife. His anxiety affected his appetite and his sleeping pattern did not improve. He said: "I became obsessed with everything". If his wife was late coming home from shopping, he was always imagining the worst and attempted to phone her several times to "check she was okay". Sometimes he would worry so much it would induce a panic attack. His in-laws confronted Joseph and told him they were annoyed at his behaviour and several rows ensued. Despite his best efforts, Joseph could not prevent his concern, even though he felt guilty at the pain he was causing.

As the impending birth grew closer Joseph was concerned about his own behaviour, which was so unlike him and he knew the impact it was starting to have on his relationship. He was praying for the birth to come early but felt nauseous at the thought of going into the labour ward. He felt he would be judged by everyone "at not being a good father".

Joseph was relieved when the birth was normal and his baby son was "perfect". This did not alleviate his fears, however, as he still worries that something traumatic may happen to his son. He knows his wife is becoming less tolerant of his behaviour, and she has told Joseph he must go to the doctor to seek help. Joseph is still contemplating this as he cannot see how a doctor can help him.

Obsessive compulsive disorder

Postnatal obsessive-compulsive disorder (OCD)

OCD usually presents during the teenage years and can affect one in fifty people with the incidence of it being familial at around 20%–35%. It is estimated that one in ten fathers will suffer from postpartum OCD.

The neuroscience

The affected part of the brain is the orbital cortex. This is responsible for rational thinking, determining what is right or wrong. In those with OCD the cortex is hyperactive, sending signals that something is wrong. Signalling is relayed to the cingulate gyrus and this creates an anxious reaction. This will not be pacified until an action is taken to rectify the error. Once this particular action is taken, the caudate nucleus intercepts and then overrides the feelings, making it easier to get on with other actions. However, occasionally the caudate nucleus function is inhibited and even when the action is 'corrected' the feeling of anxiety and 'wrong' does not diminish. Therefore, there is a constant need to repeat the irrational, repetitive behaviour. This is determined as 'brain block' (Schwartz 2000).

OCD

A study by Lensi et al. (1996) found that men who had early onset of OCD had a significantly greater history of perinatal trauma, a greater likelihood of never having been married and frequent symptoms, which include sexual, exactness and symmetry obsessions and odd rituals. Earlier research by Santangelo et al. (1994) found that complications during delivery, particularly forceps delivery, were associated with males being nine times more likely to exhibit symptoms of OCD. It was further postulated that foetal exposure to relatively high levels of coffee, cigarettes or alcohol was a predictor of OCD in those suffering from Tourette syndrome.

OCD is an anxiety disorder that presents with the symptoms of obsession, linked with a compulsive behaviour. Obsessions are described as intrusive thoughts, those that come into the mind when you least expect them and tend to dominate any other thoughts, particularly during stressful periods. These may be preceded by an idea or an image which the father is unable to dismiss, despite the fact that they may be harrowing and cause further anxiety. The thoughts are apparently subconscious, and the father feels impotent to control or stop them (Beckstein 2001).

The father may have learnt from previous experiences that the stress levels diminish if he is able to perform certain tasks. The compulsion is the behaviour in response to these thoughts. They are ritualistic and sometimes the father is compelled to perform the behaviour in order to prevent further anxiety, or situations that could increase his stress levels. Often the behaviour is completely irrational, but the compulsion or urge to act are sometimes so overwhelming the father has no choice but to execute his task. The severity of the illness can in some cases become so uncontrollable that there is a significant interference with daily life.

With insight, some fathers with mild to moderate symptoms can function normally, but for others the debilitating urges which have to be performed with regularity, can incapacitate the father's capabilities. Research by Raines et al. (2018) concluded that there were no real differences in the presentation of symptoms between the genders, but some of the dimensions were stronger in the males compared with the females.

Over 89% of parents expressed having distressing postnatal intrusive thoughts whilst nurturing their helpless infant, but although common, it is the frequency and intensity of the thoughts that differentiates normal behaviour from postnatal OCD. There is now evidence that becoming a parent can play a significant part on the themes of obsessive and compulsive behaviours amongst new mothers and fathers (Abramowitz et al. 2001, Fairbrother & Abramowitz 2007). The inflated sense of responsibility of becoming a parent, and the fear of any probability of severe harm to the infant intensifies their anxiety. Cases have been cited of fathers experiencing a rapid onset of their pre-existing OCD which coincided with either the pregnancy or birth of the first child. The study found that 60%–90% of fathers experienced intrusive thoughts of hurting either the unborn child or, as they saw it, their vulnerable infant.

These distressing thoughts of harm included the non-intentional acts of suffocating, choking or drowning, and were of such intensity over a period of time that they had a deleterious impact on their own ability to be, as they saw it, a good father. They had to make significant efforts to avoid being in situations where they would be solely responsible for the infant's care, for example, at bath time and mealtimes when they might unintentionally injure or cause damage to the child. In some cases, they were fearful that they will inadvertently sexually abuse their child. The overestimation of the threat, overwhelming guilt and despair caused by thoughts that cannot be dampened or restrained is exhausting; therefore, it is easier to neutralise the thoughts by not presenting a situation when they could occur (Abramowitz et al. 2001, Fairbrother & Abramowitz 2007).

However, the most terrifying of postnatal intrusive thoughts are not associated with an increased risk of committing harm to the infant, and there is no evidence to suggest that fathers with a history of OCD are at any risk of acting out their obsessional thoughts. The trauma is suffered by the father who has to engage in excessive avoidance tactics in order to resist or neutralise their compulsions. Ashley Curry is an advocate for raising awareness of OCD and testifies to the fact that the condition can be controlled and fathers can get well.

Story of a father with OCD 1

Nigel did not tell anyone about his obsessive behaviour even though the pressure of this pretence caused him further anxiety. He remembered driving on a country road and thought he had knocked over a cyclist. Whilst any driver might question whether they had actually done this, the idea will be dismissed the minute he looks in the rear-view mirror. For Nigel, with his existing high anxiety levels and OCD, he was convinced that the biker was lying injured in the ditch. He drove back to the scene and there was no sign. Nigel rationalised that the biker had been taken to the hospital and he drove to the nearest hospital to confirm that the biker had been admitted. They had no knowledge of the event. Nigel drove the ten miles back to the scene, checked it and retraced his route, looking out for the injured biker. This abnormal behaviour was compounded by the fact that it was 7.30 am and Nigel had his baby daughter in the back of the car. He continued to check the route looking for any sign. Although Nigel hated this behaviour because it was exhausting and almost unbearable, he had to do it. This was to his detriment, as his wife, concerned about his whereabouts phoned the police. Nigel never took his daughter in the car again.

A story of a father with OCD 2

Sam welcomed his first-born son. Sam was diagnosed with OCD in his late teens, and had managed, with medication, his condition. He did not, however, expect the intensity of his intrusive thoughts which occurred a few weeks following the birth. Sam said he sat in the nursery watching his son sleep when he suddenly had the urge to smother his son's face with the blanket. In an effort to neutralise the thoughts, Sam stepped out of the room, took deep breaths, returned but found them resuming. This happened on several occasions but each time the thoughts intensified. He had the same thoughts whilst bottle feeding his son, but this time it was about ramming the bottle into his son's mouth so hard that it would damage his gums. He knew it was time to stop that activity too.

His wife could not understand his reluctance to feed or care for his son. She became exasperated with Sam's behaviour, and they argued about his parenting role. His wife had little knowledge about his OCD and did not understand that it had been exacerbated by the birth of his son. She interpreted his behaviour as a total disregard for his parenting role. When his wife was returning to work, Sam realised he would be the sole carer and made every excuse not to be. Despite his overwhelming fears, he tried to manage his condition, unsuccessfully. He told his wife he could not cope anymore, and their relationship rapidly deteriorated until Sam realised he needed to get professional help or he would lose both his wife and his child.

Post-traumatic stress disorder

Post-traumatic Stress Disorder (PTSD) is an anxiety disorder usually caused by experiencing a frightening, distressing or terrifying event over which the individual has no control. The traumatic event is re-enacted in the mind, often in the form of flashbacks and nightmares. PTSD is marked by low, to moderate, to severe symptoms.

The neuroscience

The cause of post-traumatic stress disorder is the only major mental disorder that is now understood. One of the major pathophysiological bases for PTSD is caused by multiple molecular pathways causing an excess of excitatory signalling. Synapses are junctions which allow a neuron to electrically or chemically transmit a signal from one cell to another. They can be excitatory or inhibitory. Inhibitory synapses decrease the probability of the firing action of a potential of a cell, whilst the excitatory synapses increase its likelihood, causing a positive action in potential neurons and cells. This excess signalling within the limbic system can lead to intense emotional reactions being triggered by traumatic events. This forces the logical part of the brain to process emotional information, making it more difficult to control thoughts. There is now increasing evidence to suggest that dopamine, responsible for motivation, reward prediction and addiction, is now crucial in the regulation of fear and anxiety (Amorapanth et al. 2000, Yehuda & LeDoux 2007, Glover et al. 2011).

PTSD

Genetic studies on PTSD have been difficult, as those with a genetic risk for PTSD may not be exposed to a traumatic event. However, there is evidence which states that PTSD is heavily influenced by genetic factors, with emerging literature on genetic variations in the neurobiological systems that drive responses to trauma. In some instances, there was decreased volume of the hippocampus and greater activity in the amygdala (Gilbertson et al. 2002, Hariri et al. 2002).

PTSD is a mixture of intrusive memories of a traumatic event, avoidance of reminders of it, emotional numbing and hyperarousal. One of the most common, yet under reported causes of PTSD for fathers is witnessing a traumatic birth. It has been well documented for mothers, but it is only recently that the damaging effects to fathers have been noted. Although, the midwife will debrief both parents following a traumatic birth, often the father struggles to recover. During a traumatic birth the life of the mother and baby are often at risk. There may be copious amounts of blood, unfamiliar equipment and the drama of medical staff attempting to save life. During this situation the father feels impotent and unable to help those he should protect the most. The fear, ignorance of the surgical interventions and helplessness can elevate anxiety and even result in terror (Stramrood et al. 2013, Bradley & Slade 2011).

There have been cases of fathers who experienced repeated nightmares and negative mood swings several months following the birth of their child. They admitted to anxiety attacks and disturbed sleep patterns because they were worried their partner would become pregnant again. Some even ceased having sex as a precaution. The difficulty was being able to understand the feelings or why they occurred. The father may struggle with his emotions towards their infant, sometimes inadvertently blaming them for their partner's pain and discomfort. Currently there is no assessment process for PTSD, but as the awareness of the condition becomes more prevalent, studies into the causes and consequences are becoming more relevant.

Story of a father with PTSD

Craig was a police officer and had been with the force for seven years when his wife became pregnant. They were both delighted, but as the pregnancy progressed a few complications arose. His wife was admitted to hospital for observation a few weeks prior to the delivery of their infant. Craig heard his wife was in labour and rushed to the hospital to be with her. He gowned up and helped his wife with her breathing exercises. When the birth was imminent, Craig held his wife and assisted the young midwife and doctor with the delivery. As the baby's head emerged Craig could see there was difficulty getting the baby out. His wife had to have an episiotomy but for Craig, all he heard was his wife's haunting screams and he witnessed a lot of blood. The doctor and midwife looked 'panic stricken' and ordered Craig out of the room, but initially he refused to go. When he did concede, he left and stood outside the labour ward. He took out his phone and was constantly checking it for information, as no-one had actually explained to him what was going on. He had tried to comfort his wife, and although he wanted to assist, felt 'totally helpless', and had to watch as his wife suffered and his baby son was rushed past him to Special Care.

Craig said "I have a tough job, but did not for one second think that I would be affected by what I saw. I couldn't sleep and kept having flashbacks about the event. Even in my nightmares I felt completely useless. One day I had a panic attack and had no idea where it came from. My mate is a midwife and he was there when it happened. He said I should speak to someone about my anxiety, which I did. When I saw my GP, she was sympathetic and referred me for some therapy. I was shocked to hear my diagnosis of PTSD but it all made sense when I talked about the birth of my son. I got better, really better and now make sure that if and when my mates go into the delivery room, they are okay when they come out. I've heard it is more common that people think, but it is good to know there is hope and help out there".

Autism: Autism spectrum disorder or ASD

Autism as a condition was first recorded around the 19th century by a French physician Jean-Marc-Gaspard Itard, who described a 'wild boy' who showed several signs of autism (Lane & Pillard 1978). 'Autos' was derived from the Greek meaning 'self'. It was later defined in the early 20th century by the Swiss psychiatrist Eugene Bleuler, who viewed it as an attempt to escape from the symptoms of schizophrenia by achieving a state of deep self-absorption. Later the condition was described as a developmental disorder with a lack of affective contact (Kanner 1943). Present day concepts are transforming cultural attitudes towards autism and Asperger's, which are now termed 'Autism Spectrum Disorder' or ASD.

There has been found to be a strong genetic predisposition to ASD. Many of the genes are involved in the functioning of the neuro synapses. There tends to be spontaneous coding mutations across many genes. There is also some evidence that bipolar disorder and schizophrenia occur more frequently in families with a history of ASD.

Essentially ASD is a developmental disability which is characterised by difficulty with impaired cognitive functioning and sensory processing behaviour. This may seriously impede communication and social relationships. Around 15% of those with ASD have average or above average intelligence, 25%–35% have borderline functioning, whilst others have difficulty in all areas of functioning.

Sensory perceptions are often acute and detailed. Visually, fathers with ASD tend to have visual acuity, noticing minute details that may be overlooked or ignored by others. There is a danger they may be distracted by the minutia of an item at the expense of a more important issue. However, this trait can develop into the impressive skill of remembering complex numbers, dates or events. External auditory stimulation may also be distracting as their sensitive hearing may enable them to concentrate on sounds that can override the more significant conversations. Internal auditory stimulation, in the form of rhymes or counting, may also cause great distraction. This debilitates the father as he is unable to interpret and prioritise the stimuli around him.

There is often a strong desire to achieve what they require. This persistent, impulsive behaviour can result in repetitive touching or performing a familiar ritual. It has been likened to mimicking the same behaviours as obsessive-compulsive disorder. These actions are difficult to control and even more difficult to manage.

Abstract concepts cause great difficulty as although the father is able to cope with facts, precise details and actualities, they are unable to understand complex situations; therefore, conversations should be factual and not open to subtleties or connotations. Coupled with the symptoms is the propensity to have high levels of anxiety and those with ASD can become easily upset. This may be caused by a confrontation with an unfamiliar environment or situation.

Story of a father with ASD

Clive was an accountant with a large firm. He had high functioning ASD and was well liked in his department. His colleagues were aware of Clive's condition and took care to explain precisely what they needed and were tolerant of his idiosyncrasies. They were mindful of his inability to sense humour and were cautious not to upset him by making jokes or playing tricks.

When his wife became pregnant, Clive's family was delighted but also cautious. They were proud of Clive and the devotion he and his wife displayed towards each other. His parents decided to meet with the head of Clive's department, to discuss their thoughts on the pregnancy, birth and how Clive may react to this different situation. They all recognised the potential anxiety this would cause Clive and the pressure it could put on the marriage. Together they formulated a strategy which would pave the way for Clive to be supported in every way.

His parents told Clive they would be staying with him and his wife the week before and a few weeks following the birth to ensure the couple would be well supported. Following the birth, those who had been close to him all his life, were able to understand and manage Clive's anxieties. They ensured he was instructed at every step and that he was allowed to rest often. They were watchful for signs of anxiety and were able to prevent any escalation. A few weeks later, Clive's parents were able to return to their home. They said "Clive managed beautifully. He was magnificent. We genuinely thought he would go to pieces, but with attention to detail and correct management, he did a wonderful job and is a wonderful father".

Attention deficit hyperactivity disorder (ADHD)

This was first recognised as a valid condition in young children in the UK in 2000, but not officially recognised as an adult condition until 2008. In 1990 only forty children in the UK were on medical treatment, which means many adults had not been treated or managed properly. This resulted in many fathers either not being appropriately diagnosed with ADHD or not being diagnosed at all (Wang et al. 2017).

ADHD is characterised by inappropriate levels of activity, impulsive behaviours and lack of attention. The symptoms of ADHD are consistently related to stressful situations, though there is limited information on this. The symptoms are likely to affect parenting as stressed mothers were unable manage their infant's behaviour less successfully than those who were not stressed (Williamson & Johnston 2017).

The Diagnostic and Statistical Manual of Mental Disorders 111 (1986) initially included the diagnosis of ADHD with, or without hyperactivity. It has now become associated with global anxieties over hyperactivity (DSM 1V). It is the most common behavioural neurodevelopmental disorder and affects 5%–7% of schoolchildren. In order to be diagnosed there should be six or more disorder symptoms that have persisted for at least six months in two or more settings. Those over seventeen years of age should have at least five symptoms, prior to twelve years of age.

Most fathers may not be aware they have ADHD or have not been diagnosed until their late teens, but on reflection can determine how their thoughts, feelings influenced the way they behaved. The symptoms have to be present in two or more settings, and there should be clear evidence that they interfere with work functioning and are not explained by another mood disorder. The first symptom is inattention, which is characterised by being easily distracted, difficulty in holding attention, being careless in school or the workplace, not listening to instructions, difficulty organising tasks and activities. Other symptoms are hyperactivity and impulsivity which are portrayed as fidgeting, by tapping hands or feet, trouble taking turns, interrupting frequently or is anxious to answer, before the question is completed (Langhoff et al. 2011, Scassellati et al. 2012, Barnett 2016, Leung & Lun 2016).

Management of the condition is to improve the core symptoms of inattention, hyperactivity and impulsive behaviour. A combination of therapies combined with medication is known to affective. The most commonly used medications are stimulants, including selective norepinephrine reuptake inhibitors. These increase the activity of norepinephrine and dopamine in the prefrontal cortex, increase the activity of the extracellular concentrations of norepinephrine and dopamine at the neuronal synapse, increase the release of catecholamines from the presynaptic neurons, block reuptake of catecholamines into the presynaptic neuron, and inhibit monoamine oxidase. They have been shown to enhance behavioural and social functioning in the short term. This leads to positive self-esteem and improved parent child relationships The available catecholamines, acting as neurotransmitters, stimulate the reticular activating system, limbic system and other areas of the brain that control attention, arousal, and the inhibitory process (Devilbiss & Berridge 2008, Wilens 2008, Sudre et al. 2017).

Tricyclic antidepressants may be used where stimulants are unable to be tolerated. The medication can improve mood, impulsivity and allow the tolerance of frustration but work less well for inattention. They are, however, useful for those who suffer from depression and anxiety (Hunt et al. 2001, Leung & Lun 2016). Medication is usually superior to behavioural therapy for reducing the core symptoms of ADHD. The combination of medication and behavioural therapy was not found to be significantly more effective than medication alone (Jensen et al. 2001). Diet can also play an important part and includes the elimination of artificial colouring and flavourings, the restriction of sugar intake; however, some studies are skeptical of the benefits of such diet changes (AAP 2001, 2013, Leung & Lemay 2003).

Story of a father with ADHD

Sean was diagnosed with ADHD in his late 30s. he was unaware that he had the condition and was surprised and somewhat relieved when the physician explained why he felt as he did. He always felt that he was the naughty boy in school because he was unable to sit still and had difficulties completing his work as he was just not interested in what was being taught. However, he realised he had to make more of an effort than the others to achieve good grades in his exams.

Sean had great aspirations for his young infant daughter, but was disappointed when she failed to walk at an early age. He was even more frustrated when she failed to talk at the age of three years. He got cross with her and often made his daughter cry. She became reluctant to be with him and preferred the company of others, which made Sean even angrier. He did not realise his relationship with his daughter was deteriorating and ultimately, that of his wife. He had to seek help.

Once he was given the diagnosis and read about the consequences on the internet, Sean realised that he had to improve his parenting skills. He recognised he needed treatment as he had to fix himself before he could fix anyone or anything else. The doctor prescribed medication, which he had to take regularly. At first, he was reluctant to take them and wanted to reduce the initial dosage, but was advised against doing so. He persevered and gradually overcame the strangeness of the feelings and realised he was calmer and more in control of his life than he had ever been. Sean was a great one for sweet drinks and confectionary items and decided to reduce his intake. However, this appeared to have little effect, in fact he found the higher his caffeine intake the more he was able to sleep.

He was advised to see a counsellor to help with his anger issues and after a few months and several sessions, Sean could see how his behaviour was affecting his relationships. He worked to modify his behaviours, but more importantly explained to his wife about how and why he felt as he did. Once the medication started to work, so did Sean's relationship.

He still required help and knew that he would benefit from playing the sport he loved, but since the birth of his daughter, he had neglected it.

Sean was more attentive towards his daughter. He acknowledged that he was more important in her life than out of it and took positive steps to engage with her. He set realistic goals, as he realised that because of his ADHD, his parenting skills would be challenging. He learnt to listen, using the skills he had learnt from his counselling sessions. He attended to his daughter's strengths, and accepted what she was good at and how far she had developed. He heaped praise on her and remembered to avoid scolding her. She was gaining resilience and mastering her own independence, and Sean was instrumental in that. Sean said he was so grateful for the interventions as he was able to enjoy his daughter's upbringing and felt more fulfilled himself.

Personality disorder and borderline personality

Those diagnosed with a personality disorder are usually referred to as having a personality associated with functional impairment. It is relatively common, with approximately 5% of the population having the disorder. Their impulsive behaviour tends to deviate markedly from the norms of society and sometimes this tends to be unacceptable. Their thinking is sometimes disturbed, and they may have intense, erratic emotions which they find difficult to control. This often leads to unstable relationships coupled with the fear that they will be abandoned. Male perpetrators of domestic violence have been shown to have higher rates of personality disorder compared with non-abusive men, and their behaviour has often been associated with both general violence and intimate partner violence (Else et al. 1993, Peters et al. 2016).

The risk factors often involve a history of serious family problems, domestic violence and abuse, and severe punishments during childhood. Often the father has a history of drug misuse and depression, though personality disorders can be linked to psychosis, eating disorders and post-traumatic stress disorder.

There are several types of classification of personality disorder and include paranoia, schizoid, histrionic and dependent. To complicate the diagnosis, many may be diagnosed with several features. Of the subtypes, those with borderline and antisocial personality disorders are often known to social and medical services. The father diagnosed with a borderline personality is characterised by his volatile relationships, sometimes caused by his impulsiveness and unstable self-image. The impulsive behaviours may cause him to self-harm. The father with an antisocial personality disorder is portrayed as one who tends to break the rules, often participating in criminal behaviour. He is more likely to display intensive anger and to externalise rather than internalise his wrath. The overall demeanour is of a father who has a strong tendency to be reckless, irresponsible and deceitful (Baves & Parker 2016). Compared to women's behaviour, men with personality disorder tend to exhibit greater violence, self-harm and aggression. In one study, nearly a quarter of men engaged in severe forms of deliberate self-harm, which included cutting and swallowing dangerous substances (Gardner et al. 2016).

As more is learnt about the role of brain circuitry, genetics and neuromodulators, there is increasing understanding of the role of neurobiology in the differences and pathology in personality. The individual differences in the cognitive processes, affective reactivity, and anxiety may, in the extreme, make some more prone to a personality disorder. One study noted that impulsive aggressive behaviour may be due to excessive reactivity of the amygdala, reduced prefrontal inhibition and diminished serotonergic facilitation of the prefrontal controls (Siever & Weinstein 2009).

Unstable behaviour and the aggressive reaction to other people's emotions may be caused by excessive limbic reactivity in the brain circuits. The difficulties in processing and organising the data that the brain receives may contribute to the detached behaviour and distortions of perception. Some have a low threshold for anxiety and this may be responsible for them to enact avoidance, dependent and compulsive behaviours, which are often found in those with personality disorders (Siever & Weinstein 2009). The treatment usually relies on psychotherapeutic interventions though there is little evidence to suggest that one form of psychotherapy is more effective than another type.

Personality disorder is not as rare as is generally viewed, and research continues to uncover more robust information, however, there is still much to be learnt. Studies into the causes need to investigate both genetic and psychosocial factors which interact with the function of the neurotransmitters, which lead to cognitive and emotional regulations and traits. It is also suggested that there needs to be clearer evidence on the causes and the relationship with childhood and adolescence. It has been linked with major depression, and if there is an improvement in the personality disorder then this is followed by an improvement in the symptoms of depression, which suggests that it is important to treat the personality disorder in the first instance (Gunderson et al. 2004, Leichsenring et al. 2011).

References

Abramowitz JS, Moore KM, Carmin C, Wiegartz P, Purdon C. 2001. Obsessive-compulsive disorder in males following childbirth. *Psychosomatics*, 42, pp. 429–431.

American Academy of Pediatrics. 2001. Committee on quality improvement, subcommittee on attention-deficit/hyperactivity disorder. Clinical practice guidelines: Treatment of the school-aged child with attention deficit/hyperactivity disorder. *Pediatrics*, 108, pp. 1033–1044.

American Psychiatric Association. 1986. *Diagnostic and Statistical Manual of Mental Disorders*, 3rd ed. Washington DC: Author, p. 111.

American Psychiatric Association. 2013. *Diagnostic and Statistical Manual of Mental Disorders*, 5th ed. Arlington, VA: Author, pp. 101–105

Amorapanth P, LeDoux J, Nader K. 2000. Different lateral amygdala outputs mediate reactions and actions elicited by a fear-arousing stimulus. *Nature Neuroscience*, 3, pp. 74–79.

Barnett R. 2016. Attention deficit hyperactivity disorder. *The Lancet*, 387(10020), p. 737.

Baves A, Parker G. 2016. Borderline personality disorder in men: A literature review and illustrative case vignettes. *Psychiatric Research*, 257, pp. 197–202.

Beckstein CL. 2001. *Gender Differences in Obsessive Compulsive Disorder Symptomatology*. Michigan, USA: ProQuest Dissertations Publishing, 3018293.

Bradley R, Slade P. 2011. A review of mental health problems in fathers following the birth of a child. *Journal of Reproductive and Infant Psychology*, 29, pp. 19–42.

Devilbiss DM, Berridge CW. 2008. Cognition-enhancing doses of methylphenidate preferentially increase prefrontal cortical neuronal responsiveness. *Biological Psychiatry*, 64, pp. 626–635.

Else LT, Wonderlich SA, Beatty WW, Christie DW, Staton RD. 1993. Personality characteristics of men who physically abuse women. *Hosp Community Psychiatry*, 44(1), pp. 54–58.

Fairbrother N, Abramowitz J. 2007. New parenthood as a risk factor for the development of obsessional problems. *Behaviour Research and Therapy*, 4(9), pp. 2155–2163.

Gardner KJ, Dodsworth J, Klonsky ED. 2016. Reasons for non-suicidal self-harm in adult male offenders with and without borderline personality traits. *Archives of Suicide Research*, 20(4), pp. 614–634.

Gilbertson MW, Shenton ME, Ciszewski A et al. 2002. Smaller hippocampal volume predicts pathologic vulnerability to psychological trauma. *Nature Neuroscience*, 5, pp. 1242–1247.

Glover EM, Phifer JE, Crain DF, Norrholm SD, Davis M, Bradley B, Ressler KJ, Jovanovic T. 2011. Tools for translational neuroscience: PTSD is associated with heightened fear responses using acoustic startle but not skin conductance measures. *Depression and Anxiety*, 28, pp. 1058–1066.

Glover V. 2014. Maternal depression, anxiety and stress during pregnancy and child outcome; what needs to be done. *Best Practice and Research Clinical obstetrics and Gynaecology*, 28(1), pp. 25–35.

Gunderson JG, Moreym LC, Stout RL et al. 2004. Major depressive disorder and borderline personality disorder revisited: Longitudinal interactions. *Journal of Clinical Psychiatry*, 65, pp. 1049–1056.

Hariri AR, Mattay VS, Tessitore A et al. 2002. Serotonin transporter genetic variation and the response of the human amygdala. *Science*, 297, pp. 400–403.

Hunt RD, Paquin A, Payton K. 2001. An update on assessment and treatment of complex attention-deficit hyperactivity disorder. *Pediatric Annals*, 30(3), pp. 162–172.

Kanner L. 1943. Autistic disturbances of affective contact. *Nervous Child*, 2, pp. 217–250.

Lane H, Pillard R. 1978. *The Wild Boy of Burundi: The Story of an Outcast Child*. Manhattan, New York, USA: Random House Publishers.

Langhoff J, Kesmodel U, Jacobsson B, Rasmussen S, Vogel I. 2006. Spontaneous preterm delivery in primiparous women at low risk in Denmark: Population based study. *BMJ*, 332(5747), pp. 937–939.

Leichsenring F, Leibing E, Kruse J, New AS, Leweke F. 2011. Borderline personality disorder. *The Lancet*, 377(9759), pp. 74–84.

Lensi P, Cassano GB, Correddu G, Ravagli S. 1996. Obsessive–compulsive disorder: Familial–developmental history, symptomatology, comorbidity and course with special reference to gender-related differences. *BMJ*, 169(1), pp. 101–107.

Leung AK, Lemay JF. 2003. Attention deficit hyperactivity disorder: An update. *Advances in Therapy*, 20, pp. 305–318.

Leung AKC, Lun K. 2016. Attention-deficit/hyperactivity disorder. *Advances in Pediatric's*, 63, pp. 255–280.

Markowitsch HJ, Staniloiu A. 2011. Amygdala in action: Relaying biological and social significance to autobiographical memory. *Neuropsychologia*, 49(4), pp. 718–733.

Morgan V, Pickens D, Gautam S, Kessler R, Mertz H. 2005. Amitriptyline reduces rectal pain related activation of the anterior cingulate cortex in patients with irritable bowel syndrome. *Gut*, 54(5), pp. 601–607.

Peters JR, Derefinko KJ, Lynam DR. 2016. Negative urgency accounts for the association between borderline personality features and intimate partner violence in young men. *Journal of Personality Disorder*, 31(1), pp. 16–25.

Raines AM, Oglesby ME, Allan NP, Mathes BM, Sutton C, Schmidt N. 2018. Examining the role of sex differences in obsessive compulsive symptom dimensions. *Psychiatry Research*, 259, pp. 265–269.

Rubertsson C, Hellström J, Cross M, Sydsjö G. 2014. Anxiety in early pregnancy: Prevalence and contributing factors. *Archives of Women's Mental Health*, 17(3), pp. 221–228.

Santangelo SL, Pauls DL, Goldstein JM, Faraone SV, Tsuang MT, Leckman J. 1994. Tourette's syndrome: What are the influences of gender and comorbid obsessive-compulsive disorder? *Journal of the American Academy of Child and Adolescent Psychiatry*, 33(6), pp. 795–804.

Scassellati C, Bonvicini C, Faraone SV et al. 2012. Biomarkers and attention-deficit/hyperactivity disorder: A systematic review and meta-analysis. *Journal of the American Academy of Child and Adolescent Psychiatry*, 51, pp. 1003–1019.

Schwartz JM. 2000. *Brain Lock*. New York, USA: Regan Publishers.

Siever LJ, Weinstein LN. 2009. The neurobiology of personality disorders: Implications for psychoanalysis. *American Journal of Psychoanalysis*, 57(2), pp. 361–398.

Stramrood C, Doornbos B, Wessel I, Geenen M, Asrnoudse J, Berg P, Weijmar SW, Pampus M. 2013. Fathers with PTSD and depression in pregnancies complicated by preterm preeclampsia or PPROM. *Archives of Gynecology and Obstetrics*, 2879(4), pp. 635–661.

Stuebe AM, Grewen K, Pedersen CA, Propper C, Meltzer-Brody S. 2012. Failed lactation and perinatal depression: Common problems with shared neuroendocrine mechanisms? *Journal of Women's Health*, 2(3), pp. 264–272.

Sudre G, Szekely E, Sharp W et al. 2017. Multimodal mapping of the brain's functional connectivity and the adult outcome of attention deficit hyperactivity disorder. *Proceedings of the National Academy of Sciences of the United States of America*, 114(44), pp. 11787–11792.

Wang LJ, Lee SY, Yuan SS, Yang CJ, Yang KC, Huang TS, Chou WJ, Chou MC, Lee MJ, Lee TL, Shyu YC. 2017. Prevalence rates of youths diagnosed with and medicated for ADHD in a nationwide survey in Taiwan from 2000 to 2011. *Epidemiology and Psychiatric Sciences*, 26(6), pp. 624–634.

WHO. 2018. International Classification of Diseases 11th Revision (ICD 11). https://www.who.int/news-room/detail/18-06-2018-who-releases-new-international-classification-of-diseases-(icd-11), accessed 18 October 2019.

Wilens TE. 2008. Effects of methylphenidate on the catecholaminergic system in attention-deficit/hyperactivity disorder. *Journal of Clinical Psychopharmacology*, 28, pp. S46–S53.

Williamson D, Johnston C. 2017. Maternal ADHD symptoms and parenting stress: The roles of parenting self-efficacy beliefs and neuroticism. *Journal of Attention Disorders*, 23(5), pp. 493–505.

Yehuda R, LeDoux J. 2007. Response variation following trauma: A translational neuroscience approach to understanding PTSD. *Neuron*, 55(1), pp. 19–32.

Chapter 4

The types of conditions

Depression

The changes in lifestyle, the challenges and adjustments to a new member of the family can present as an equally stressful time for the father as well as the mother. There is now sufficient evidence to say that this stress during the ante- and postnatal period can also lead to depression in the father. A study by Fletcher et al. in (2006) found that around 2%–5% of new fathers were diagnosed with depression, though the prevalence rate has varied widely with some figures rising, with one in ten being quoted by several sources (Paulson & Bazemore 2011, Cameron et al. 2015). Reviews found that there was a strong link to the father suffering from depression during the postnatal period if his partner also had moderate to severe postnatal depression (Goodman 2004, Schumacher et al. 2008).

The lack of funding for sufficiently large randomised controlled studies, differences in the presentation of the illness, treatment strategies and the complexities of the brain structure have all compromised the reasons for the scarcity of significant research into mental illness. The explanation for the causes of depression and depressive symptoms are rudimentary, but with adequate resources, greater progress and insights are possible.

The neuroscience

Recent scientific discoveries have given significant weight to the facts that depression is not a lifestyle choice nor a sign of weakness, but a neurological condition. It presents as a set of neuroanatomical structures in the prefrontal lobe and the limbic areas of the brain, which are involved in affective regulation. The alterations in the activities of these structures influences the way in which the brain functions and how this has implications for the origins of depressive disorders.

Investigative neuroscientists are uncovering the ways in which the brain's chemicals work and the differing incidents in depressed and anxious people. They have examined the structural, functional and molecular alterations which occur in several areas of the brain and have explored the role of glucocorticoids, inflammatory cytokines, genetic components and the alterations of the grey matter of the brain (El-Sayed et al. 2012).

It has long been believed that depression and other mental disorders and illness are as a result of a chemical imbalance within the brain. It is postulated that one of the reasons for depression is caused by an imbalance of neurotransmitters, primarily serotonin and dopamine, a lack of which is associated with the feelings of pleasure and gratification. However, its biological function is complex and multifaceted as it is responsible for modulating cognition, reward, learning and memory amongst other physiological processes (Young 2007).

Epigenetics

Work on epigenetics is uncovering the impact of different gene variations. People who have the variation in the gene that codes for a serotonin receptor, called 5-HTT, are more likely to be susceptible to depression following a stressful life event than those who do not present with the mutation. This mutation reduces the production of the number of serotonin receptors in the brain which, in turn, causes a decrease in serotonin signalling. There is also evidence to suggest that there are changes in the dopamine signalling in the brain (Holloway T & Gonzalez-Maeso 2015).

The advances of brain magnetic resonance (MRI) and CAT scans have allowed scientists to examine what happens within the brains of people who are mentally ill. Brain imaging studies have found that those with depression have less grey matter in several areas of the brain, particularly the cortex, hippocampus and the amygdala. Grey matter contains the cell bodies, dendrites, ganglia and axon terminals of neurons and is where all synapses are located and therefore where all the signalling occurs. These changes can affect emotions, memory and decision making. This suggests that depression is as likely to be caused by the brain structure than the actual neuro chemicals.

It has also been found that the plasticity of the hippocampus, an area of the brain responsible for memory and emotion, shrinks in people with recurrent and poorly treated depression (Schmaal et al. 2015). This means that making choices and the general ability to take care of personal day to day living is very limited, and it is difficult to recover from feelings of despair. This may be due to changes in the brain's plasticity which allows neurons to change their signalling in response to new information, and it is possible that it is responsible for the reduction in the growth of new brain cells, or neurogenesis. Therefore, it is thought that chronic stress has a negative impact on the brain's plasticity.

Studies have linked depression to the immune system and have noted the co-prevalence of depression with vascular and inflammatory disorders; in inflammation this is associated with reduced levels of serum albumin and zinc (Dantzer 2009, Maes et al. 2012). Inflammatory disorders have also been associated with alterations in behaviour. It has been suggested that there are links to the immune system as depressed people have unusually high levels of cytokines. These are small proteins which play a part in the inflammation process, released during an infection.

Symptoms are characterised by pyrexia, lethargy, sleep and appetite disturbances (Hart 1988). The high levels of cytokines are usually caused by stress and can impact normal neurotransmitter signalling, which then leads to the symptoms of depression. With this new information, anti-inflammatory drugs are sometimes prescribed, together with antidepressants.

Baumeister et al. (2016) found that people who had experienced traumatic events or severe stress during childhood had higher levels of brain inflammation in adulthood. This knowledge, and the need for further information in what is a complex subject, suggest that inflammation and the individual components of cytokines, associated genes and their interaction with environmental factors are now the focus of future research.

Fathers have a biological response to fatherhood and are at a higher risk of being depressed postnatally if their testosterone levels decrease nine months following the birth of their infant. Low testosterone levels during this time may be normal and act as a natural adaption to parenthood. It may also affect the mother as she tended to have fewer depressive symptoms nine to fifteen months following the birth. Fathers with high levels of testosterone had a greater risk of being stressed and hostile towards their partner (Saxbe et al. 2017).

Presentation of depression

There are several features to paternal depression, most of which are familiar to both genders. The symptoms of maternal postnatal depression are well documented, but those attributed to men, although similar, are often presented differently. The profound and consistent lowering of his mood state explains why his emotional responses are at their slowest, and it is difficult for him to summon up any energy or enthusiasm. The father may lack energy and have to be coerced into doing things, which he may reluctantly perform. Designated male tasks, to include washing the car or mowing the lawn may be neglected and with these omissions, the overall care of the household suffers. This can be frustrating for the mother who relied on the support of her partner to help with the care of the infant.

Social activities may be avoided as any interaction with his mates, may expose him to ridicule and or unwanted sympathy. Although friends may be sympathetic towards him, they often cannot exhibit the empathetic responses the father may need or require. The father may be aware that he is feeling sad and really 'down' and feel like crying, but social conditioning determines that this is not possible, even in this enlightened age. It is probable that a man crying in public, after the initial shock, will promote embarrassment and sometimes ridicule.

With the slowing down of the father's psychomotor functioning, thoughts are sluggish and may result in thought-blocking where he is unable to realise his thought processes and cease his dialogue during mid-sentence. Responding to questions may be difficult as it may be challenging to assimilate what has been said, let alone formulate an answer. This can be interpreted as ignorance or avoidance and could possibly be met with aggression from his partner. This might be seen as a lack of understanding of his condition, and the reaction is one of equal aggression.

As noticed in a previous chapter, the care of his infant may be compromised, particularly if the father's depression is severe. His lack of concentration, together with his poor functioning may lead to the false belief that his infant is unable to respond to him because his paternal skills are deficient. This may be exacerbated if the infant cries and cannot be placated by him, but can be placated by others, neglecting to understand that his own emotions are being transferred to his infant. In extreme cases, the care of the infant may be neglected, particularly if the father is the main carer, because he is too ill to concentrate on feeding regimes or have the energy to change nappies. Guilt can exacerbate the problem and the lack of insight from others deepens the anger. Comparisons may be made between the life pre and post infant, and the reason for the decline in the father's mental health is clearly the fault of the infant. It is possible this will result in irritation with the infant and anger at his partner.

A healthy diet is often a secondary need as the father's appetite is compromised. There may be fluctuations in weight gain or loss because of the irregular mealtimes. Sometimes this may be his fault or the fault of the infant's demands. It is not unusual for the effort of making a meal to be overwhelming, making snacking the preferred option. For some fathers it can be preferable to eat out or pick up fast food than be expected to cook for the family. Comfort eating with sweet, high calorific value foods, eaten as an antidote to the depression, can cause an increase in weight, whilst forgoing food altogether in favour of drinking alcohol can cause weight loss. He may neglect going to the gym, possibly a full-time occupation, for all the reasons outlined above. This lack of exercise can result in weight gain and intensify his poor mood state. The erratic diet and lack of exercise can result in a disturbance of bowel movements, manifesting as either constipation, loose stools or a combination of both.

Sleep deprivation, caused by his depression, not his infant's night time demands, contributes to his emotional affrays and has implications for his performance at work and home. In extreme, sometimes unrecognised cases, the father's mood may be so low that he feels his only option for respite is to resort to suicide. However, there is still stigma attached to the act of suicide, as referenced by the previous term 'to commit suicide' which was an unlawful act. Some men believe that suicide may be seen as a sign of weakness or selfishness for their family's future and wellbeing. As a result, they may resort to the more insidious approach of faking accidental death by either driving recklessly or combining drinking alcohol and taking drugs rather than be known as having died through 'suicide'. The possibility must never be discounted, and it is important that suicide ideation is always addressed. Once recognised there has to be a sound knowledge of how to prevent suicide occurring (WHO 2016).

Finally, and probably firstly, his libido is reduced. Brice Pitt wrote that 'in depression, libido is the first thing to go, and in recovery, the first thing to come back'. This may be of some comfort to the father, but often the reasons why sex life has deteriorated is misconstrued as the father not being sexually attracted to his partner or that he has found another love interest. It is rarely attributed to depression (Pitt 1993).

Several factors may contribute to the father's condition. An unsupported relationship or where the mother is unable to be compassionate because she is suffering from a mental disorder herself, can have a significant impact on the health of the father. The relationship might have already been strained, and the added pressures of the infant can compound the poor communication that may have been a previous problem. A diminishing sex life will also have consequences for mental health in both persons. Some evidence has pointed out that fathers who expected their sex life to continue, or even increase following the birth, were disillusioned at the decrease in intimacy within their relationship. It has been suggested that there is may be a mutual attraction to a partner's psychosocial state and therefore they are more likely to form a relationship (Deater-Deckard et al. 1998).

The unrealistic expectations and a lack of awareness or education about the process of child care and the pressures that it brings, may emphasise the resentment he feels. This may leave him susceptible to criticism and as a result may further compound any lack of self-esteem (Buist et al. 2003). Conversely, the fathers who were well informed about the role of the father and parenting appear to have heightened self-esteem.

The father's previous coping mechanisms may be poor. Studies have shown that if the father has difficulty coping with any adverse effect of the pregnancy or the birth itself, then he is less likely to have the appropriate strategies to cope in the postnatal period, which may ultimately lead to anxiety or depressive disorders (Johnson & Baker 2004).

The father may feel he is unable to ask for help from relatives and friends as this will not appeal to his macho image of being the provider. Extended and nuclear families are no longer as dominant as in past years, and there is no guarantee that his own mother will be available for support as she may be working or living too far away to be of assistance. There is some evidence to suggest that a poor relationship with his own mother will also affect how he will ask for help. This may also apply to his father, who may not be familiar with the needs of his son or aware of the new phenomenon of paternal depression. Some research highlighted that men in stepfamilies whose partners were single mothers had higher levels of depressive symptoms than those whose partners came from the traditional nuclear family (Deater-Deckard et al. 1998). This coupled with the lack of any further outside social and or emotional support can leave the father feeling isolated and vulnerable (Matthey et al. 2000, Boyce et al. 2007).

The father may have a history of anxiety and or depression and as the research shows, his illness can be exacerbated by the demands of the perinatal period (Matthey et al. 2000). A further complication is that the feelings of depression are sometimes so insidious, it is difficult for him to interpret how he is really feeling and his fall into the depths of despair may be unregulated (Matthey et al. 2000).

Environmental factors may also be compounders. Studies have found the impact of poor or inadequate housing prior to the birth have an impact on mental health (Evans et al. 2003). Previous issues with housing may not have been resolved and result in further overcrowding or limited space either in or outside the property. Multi-occupancy can lead to poor mental health (Barratt et al. 2015). The increasing number of gang-related crimes has been associated with poor parenting and absent fathers. The argument is that the lack of a role model can lead to low self-esteem and ultimately depression. The father may find respite joining with groups with similar interests, albeit crime related (Brennen 2018).

The father may be unemployed or on low wages and relying on benefits. The reality of the necessary expenditure for the infant will impact the already stretched family finances. If the father has been struggling to meet the needs of his workplace, a sparse finance situation may be exacerbated because of his response to the demands of his infant's needs. Most employers are sympathetic towards the new father and make exceptions for their tiredness and lateness, but this might not be the case for some employers, particularly when the impact of austerity affects the company.

It is possible that the rates of depression in fathers are underestimated because of their reticence to seek help either because they fail to recognise or they deny their disorder. The lack of assessment with screening tools and the appropriateness of them may lead to misdiagnosis or mismanagement. Depression appears to have legitimate chemical causes with a neurological underpinning, which makes the ability to overcome the illness more complicated than that of 'getting a grip'. Depression as a whole presents as a complex, multidimensional and insidious disorder, which is gradually being understood, but the onset can be attributed to genetics, epigenetics, inflammation, brain characteristics and lived experiences. When the functioning is fully understood, it may unlock the mysteries of the human consciousness.

Story of a father with depression

Mac didn't think men could suffer postnatal depression until he saw a programme about men and postnatal depression on the television. He said that he totally felt the same and could relate to all of the issues that were being discussed. Mac admitted to drinking and smoking heavily to combat his anxiety and depression which was never an issue before having a baby with his girlfriend.

He honestly felt his relationship wasn't the strongest as the pregnancy was totally unexpected, which was a blow as they were going to go travelling together for a year. Now he feels trapped, angry and in a job to provide for the family that wasn't in the plan.

Mac said: 'I hate to say this but I just have no feeling for my daughter and can easily run away but sometimes feel I will let her down in life as my parents were never really there for me due to their work. I have this fear for the next eighteen years I will be just existing not living. I'm so anxious and feeling more depressed by the day looking for any kind of happiness. I'm starting to think my girlfriend planned this without asking me or I'm feeling paranoid but sometimes it all does not add up'.

My personality totally changed. I was worried that Social Services would be involved if I owned up to my own struggles. I tried to be the man and father that I was expected to be and didn't tell my girlfriend as I did not want to make her mental health any worse. I started to avoid situations by overworking and kept myself away from my family. I made excuses not to go to any visits to my relations and said I had to go out whenever the family came over. This was just not like me as before we had our baby, I was very sociable, was the life and soul of the party, cracked jokes which my girlfriend really enjoyed. I used to love sex but avoided as I didn't want to get my girlfriend pregnant and go through the same hell again and this made me feel even worse, as a man. I looked after myself, ate good food, now I was overeating, just rubbish food and started smoking after giving up five years previously. I used to love exercising and had plenty of energy, now all I wanted to do was sleep and just sit in the chair staring at the television but not really taking anything in.

Having seen the programme, it was a real-life changer as I could see that other men had gone through the same as me. I was so relieved I looked more online and discovered someone who specialised in the same area. I emailed them and several telephone conversations later, discovered I could get well, as long as I had help and support. It took me a long time but it was really worth it as I now have a much better relationship with my partner and have got to really love my daughter.

Suicide ideation

Suicidal thoughts vary in associated risk for suicidal behaviour, and suicidal thinking at any level of intent should not be dismissed as trivial musings (Kerr et al. 2008). Suicide is a complex phenomenon, involving interactions among many different biological, psychological and social factors. Behavioural symptomology, however, provides a clearer case for recognising depressive symptoms, coupled with the risk factors and type of lifestyle.

Sometimes the emotional turmoil and pain is so overwhelming the father may feel his only recourse is to end, not only his suffering, but that of his family. He may have convinced himself that he is a burden on the family, they would be better off without him and suicide is the only option. He may plan it meticulously, in some cases, ensuring it is not an obvious suicide but could be construed as an accident. This, to ensure his family does not suffer the guilt or anger that suicide often engenders or, because it is not always clear if some insurance companies will 'cover' suicides. Sometimes the suicide is spontaneous and irrational. Whatever the method, the devastation on the family is incalculable, but equally the father must have been feeling such despair that he saw it as his only release.

The importance of preventing suicide cannot be over emphasised, and it is predominately a male disorder. It is recognised as the biggest killer of men aged between twenty and forty-nine years of age (ONS 2015). Male suicide accounts for approximately three quarters of all suicides in the UK (ONS 2018). In a study by Quevedo et al. (2011) it was established that the prevalence of the risk of suicide in fathers in the postnatal period was around 5%. Those fathers who suffered with depression were over twenty times more likely to be suicidal, whilst those who had a dual or mixed diagnosis had the propensity of an almost forty-seven times higher chance of attempting suicide than those who did not suffer from any mood disorder. This is greater than the number of men killed in road accidents, cancer and coronary heart disease. A further risk factor are the men who are subjected to the poorest socioeconomic circumstances, as they are ten times more likely to kill themselves than those in the more affluent areas (Sun & Zhang 2016).

It was found that men's reporting of suicidal behaviour was significantly higher than their partners when they were screened with the Edinburgh Postnatal Depression Scale. Evidence has shown that only 23% of men would see a GP if they felt low for more than two weeks. This is compared to 33% of women, which is still a relatively low number. One study reported substance use, depressive symptoms, and, to a limited extent, their parents' depressive symptoms were significant predictors of risk for suicidal ideation occurrence and recurrences.

Risk factors and warning signs for suicidal ideation

Expressed thoughts and feelings often provide key warning signs. Sometimes the father may talk openly about death or convey his thoughts about dying, occasionally making reference to suicidal threats and suggest that he would not be missed if he went away and perhaps, the family would be better off without him. There is often the suggestion of a sense of despair with little hope for the future and expression of negative prospects of life. However, as the father may be more discreet about his thoughts and emotions, it is important to observe any changes in behaviour.

These changes may be quite drastic, with noticeable changes over a short period of time. The father may increasingly isolate himself giving the reason that he recognises how he is viewed socially and how his intentions are misunderstood. The father acknowledges that he is becoming a burden and sees little point in talking about it. Social media may provide a platform for writing abstractly about death and dying, to the point that it becomes an obsession.

An unusually organised trait, which is illustrated by the father creating space in his and his partner's room, tidying away possessions and giving away personal objects, often which have sentimental and substantial value, is a clue to the father's intention to end his life, but also to ensure that others have mementos of him.

The father may fear the thought of death but accept it is a necessary evil. This may increase his anger and he may become increasingly irritated, resulting in morbid aggression and perhaps an increase in self- harming behaviours. He may engage in risk-taking behaviours and is oblivious of the fact he is jeopardising his life. Hoarding or escalating the amount of medication taken are also factors, whereas acquiring a lethal weapon is a clear indication of suicidal ideation. Sometimes the clues are not obvious and it is difficult to believe that a man could take his own life without anyone being aware, but it does happen.

Self-harm

Self-harm itself usually occurs in late childhood and is used as a relief from mental anguish. Self-harm has often been misunderstood as attention-seeking behaviour, which is sometimes not tolerated, as any treatment for self-inflicted injuries is seen as a waste of valuable health service resources.

However, it is more common than is thought with over 10% of adolescents admitting to a form of self-harm. Most young people reported that they started to hurt themselves around the age of twelve years. There are several myths surrounding the reasons why self-harm is prevalent, and these include that the person must belong to a specific cult which encourages this as a badge of honour—it is an enjoyable pursuit, it is exclusively girls who do it or those who self-harm have suicidal ideation (Klonsky, & Muehlenkamp 2007). There is also the stereotypical ideation of the adolescent from a low-income background, but studies have identified that many young people who self-harm can be perfectionists and high achievers who place undue pressure on themselves and feel that whatever they do is never good enough (Young 2007).

Self-harm is described as a behaviour which causes injury or harm to themselves. The most common forms are cutting, burning with naked flames or cigarettes or non-lethal overdoses of medication. For young boys and men, the most common form of self-harm is risk-taking behaviour by consuming large quantities of alcohol, driving at dangerous speeds or engaging in sexual activities without taking adequate precautions (Klonsky & Muehlenkamp 2007, Hawton et al. 2012).

It is easy to conceal some forms of self-harm by wearing long sleeves to hide scars on the arms or being fully dressed even in the warmest weather to mask bodily injuries. Sometimes tattoos may be used to disguise scars, whereas the reasons for having mass tattoos can also be a form of self-harm. The signs are often cyclical whereby the distressing thoughts can manifest into distressing feelings such as self-doubt and lacking in self-esteem. This promotes an emotional pain that is often hard to cope with, causing an emotional overload, which in itself becomes increasingly difficult to bear. Rather than suffer the despair, the physical pain felt by a cut or burn can temporarily negate the emotional pain. This relief, and the reasons behind it, can manifest as a shameful act and this can compound the distressing thoughts. Any form of self-harm should be taken seriously.

There are complexities in any form of self-harm, and reasons may be multifactorial, but studies have shown that anxiety, depression, borderline personality disorders and eating disorders are all significant factors. Social indicators may include a young person within the care system or having voluntarily left a care home. Difficulty with sexual identification is a recognised factor within the LGBT community.

Story of a father who self-harmed

Steven had been in care since the death of his father. His mother was an alcoholic and social services said she was incapable of looking after her son, and at the age of five years he was cared for by his grandmother. Steven was, by his admission, a difficult child and his grandmother often scolded him, punishing him by not giving him food until he behaved. He remembered going for days without anything to eat. He was angry with his grandmother and said he used to beat his head with his fists to try and make himself behave, but whatever he did, did not please her. Later he believed it was because she resented Steven being alive instead of her son. His behaviour and weight loss were noted by the school and a visit from the social worker ascertained that his grandmother was unable cope with him and at the age of seven years, Steven was taken into foster care, where he remained until he was twelve. During that time, he continued to hurt himself, now banging his head against the wall and slamming his shoulders into the doors. Steven remembered the first time he started smoking at the age of ten years and the pleasure he took slowly pressing the lit cigarette against his skin. Somehow it cleared his brain and he was not angry for that moment. He found just as much pleasure in slicing into his skin with the kitchen knife. He became skilled at hiding his arms and began to find that he was equally able to conceal a razorblade and that just nicking his skin on his upper arms was just as satisfying.

His girlfriend was pregnant when they were both sixteen years old. They rented a flat together in the town and when he was seventeen, he was the father to a premature daughter.

Steven said: 'I was often accused of trying to commit suicide when I used a sharp blade to cut along my forearms. They said it was only a matter of time before I cut into my main artery and then I would be dead – which is what I wanted after all. I couldn't get them to understand that I didn't want to die. This was different. I hated the way I felt and was so guilty about wanting to be away from all of this, but I had to cope with my life somehow and honestly putting that knife to my arm reminded me that there were worst things in life. My brain would stop banging away with these stupid thoughts about me. How I was a waste of time. How I needed to get a grip and how I didn't know how or what to do to get a grip. My baby daughter needed me but when she was crying in her cot, I just sat staring at the knife. One slash and I immediately felt better, and I thought I will never do this again, but I knew deep down that I would'.

It would appear that men are taught to externalise their emotions and that being more honest or open about the ability to self-harm is seen not as a problem but more as a masculine trait. Studies have shown that males are more inclined to be more open about their injuries, and tend to make larger, deeper cuts on their skin than those seen in women.

In some instances, it was more acceptable for men to conduct violent acts upon their bodies. There have been cases of men inflicting secondary harm on themselves. What is becoming more common are 'accidents' whereby the bike rider purposefully crashes the bike in order to inflict non-life threating injury, which may include grazes or fractures. Car crashes and high-risk sports, for example, snow boarding can have equal consequences if the father commits his desire to self-harm.

It is socially acceptable for a man to get drunk with a group of friends, and the more alcohol that could be tolerated, the manlier he is perceived by his fellow drinkers, even though that consumption is self-harming. The more obvious the self-harm, the less likelihood of being challenged. This belief is reinforced by the male role models portrayed in the media who convert their distress and frustration into anger by punching walls, shouting and getting into fights, eventually turning the anger on themselves. The role model can be extended to peers' behaviour, whereby self-harming can be interpreted a behaviour that should be imitated to gain a rite of passage (Adler & Adler 2011). This was evident during the 1980s 'miners' strike', when the frustration felt by the miners was transferred to their violent behaviour in the football crowds. The mining working population was affected by mine closures, causing loss of work, stress and depression. At this time, it was noted that there was an increase in violent behaviour within football crowds.

Any concern about changes in the father's emotional state or changes in his behaviour, should be addressed. It is important to understand why he feels like this. Listening is a skill and hearing someone talk about death is disturbing; but he deserves to be listened to and all the warning signs taken seriously. A man who has expressed a potential suicide threat should never be left alone but accompanied until medical help arrives, or accompanied to the general practitioner.

Bipolar disorder

Bipolar disorder was previously known as manic-depression and often was described as the circle of insanity. The German psychiatrist Kraepelin outlined manic depressive illness and recognised the influence of the brain to cause severe shifts in mood function.

This terminology changed in 1980, to Bipolar Disorder following the publication of the third edition of the Diagnostic and Statistical Manual of Mental Disorders (DSM3). It presents as a conflict or change in the mood status of the father. One day he can be full of the joys of spring, expressing a positive outlook on life, whilst the next day he can be wallowing in the realms of despair. That of course is an over simplification of the condition as the variants of mood can rapidly change over a few hours. This inability to predict the father's emotions, coupled with impossible behaviour, often leads to confusion, irritation and exasperation because it is difficult to understand what is really going on. It is also difficult for the father to understand his mental condition, and it is not uncommon for him to disguise his symptoms. There is extensive evidence to confirm that fathers, in particular, will not admit to being depressed and will take exceptional measures to avoid any identification of their mental state. It is postulated that the symptoms of depression defy the male notion of independence and emotional control (Pipich & Shrand 2018).

Until recently, the condition was poorly understood and the dramatic shifts of untreated mood swings often caused a treatment dilemma. To compound the problem one feature of bipolar disorder is that it can lay dormant, and the father may have extended periods when he will be mentally well, making the illness more difficult to predict. It is recognised that bipolar disorder can be deeply disruptive and have a damaging impact on functionality and quality of life.

The symptoms often develop during late adolescence or early adulthood. When one parent has bipolar disorder, the risk to each child is 15%–30%. When both parents have bipolar disorder, the risk increases to 50%–75%. The risk of siblings and fraternal twins is 15%–25%. The risk in identical twins is approximately 70%. Current statistics put it at around 2.6% of the male population age eighteen and over. A significantly high number of intelligent people have been found to be suffering from bipolar disorder. Studies have shown that men tend to develop bipolar disorder at an earlier age than women and their first episode usually presents as a manic episode. Their symptoms tend to have a greater severity and they appear to be more prone to more manic episodes than women (Arnold 2003). It is possible for the condition to be misdiagnosed and is only really reliable following a clear-cut episode of mania. It is often misdiagnosed as attention deficit disorder.

Genetic component

Although there is a genetic predisposition to bipolar disorder, it is not necessarily the case that everyone with an inherited vulnerability will develop the condition. This is a strong indicator that other, external factors may influence behaviour. In order to develop a greater understanding of the efficacy of treatments and how they may be improved, currently there is a large-scale study, the *Australian Genetics of Bipolar Disorder Study,* which aims to identify the genes that predispose people to bipolar disorder and responses to medication. This opens up interesting terrain and suggests that in the future it may be possible to screen a foetus for the gene.

The signs of mania are the opposite of those experienced during a depressive phase. In mania the father's thoughts may be rapid and his mood euphoric, imaging everything that he would like to achieve in a torrent of ideas, but unable to have the capacity or competence to complete them. The reality is that the father feels, often for no particular reason, supremely confident, exhilarated and generally wonderful. This air of being in control makes the disorder difficult to detect, particularly where confidence is synonymous with his masculinity (Pipich & Shrand 2018).

Conversely, should the father recognise that he has failed to impress then he will make every effort to be convincing, with even more bizarre ideas. Perhaps frustrated with any lack of interest or perceived barriers, this will only lend to increase his determination to make it work. In an effort to get fit, this may include going online to book an exotic holiday, order an expensive pair of trainers to help him run the marathon, purchase numerous seeds to start a vegan vegetable patch or place a ridiculously large bet on a horse to fund his campaign. This irrational, risk-taking behaviour can and often leads to the father going into debt. These feelings of exhilaration often alienate and exhaust family and friends. This is compounded by the fact that this is the time when the mother of his infant needs him at his most rational, responsible and caring.

On the converse side, any attempt at communicating ineffectively can cause him to become irritated, miserable and may sometimes manifest as aggressive behaviour, and it is more likely that he will injure himself or others during the manic phase because of arguing, shouting, and or fighting. This can lead to admission to hospital or being arrested for inappropriate behaviour. His inability to concentrate on one subject often means he can be easily distracted. The augmented intensity of instability and the frequency of the alteration of mood can be deeply distressing and complicates any recognition of the disorder and as a result can impede the treatment process.

When the father's mood swings into the depressive phase, this mimics the signs and symptoms described in the section on depression. It is important to understand that there is evidence to suggest there is a high risk of suicide ideation in men with bipolar disorder with a greater rate of male suicides.

There is no doubt that during the manic phase the father's energy levels cause him to be constantly active, with periods where he will be incapable of resting. During this phase a heightened sense of sexuality is common. Hypersexuality is often a precursor of a manic episode and is described as a dysfunctional preoccupation with sexual behaviours or fantasies which are difficult to control. This can include impulsive, reckless sexual behaviours where the father may experience poor judgement in his advances to his partner or other women. This is not always the case, but studies have found that men experiencing bipolar disorder claim to notice a difference in their behaviour during the manic phase as they constantly think about sex, are more interested in pornography, make constant sexual demands on their partner or may result in infidelity with multiple one-night stands with multiple partners (Kopeykina et al. 2016).

Once the condition is recognised, treated and under control, the feelings dissipate, and men will often regret and be remorseful of their previous actions. If left untreated it has serious consequences for the unbearable strain it imposes on sexual relationships and can lead to breakdown in communication, as it is reported that couples who experience bipolar disorder suffer from decreased levels of sexual satisfaction. As with depressive symptoms, it is important to ascertain whether he intends to or has any ideas about harming himself, and if so, what does he intend to do about this and to what extent is he prepared to carry it out.

Self-medication

The lack of insight or control hampers the father's ability to understand when his feelings of euphoria are a blessing or a curse. He is safe in the knowledge that medication can easily and effectively numb any surges of creativity. It would seem unreasonable to permanently destroy his mood when a glass of whiskey can temporarily disarm him. The same might be said for a joint of cannabis, a line of cocaine. The delusion that he can achieve anything he wants to, however unrealistic, can be enhanced by the temporary 'lift' which spurs on his creativity or boosts his thought processes. When exhaustion hits, the inability to rest or sleep becomes problematic, and it is therefore a must to seek out a drink or drug which is capable of quieting their mind. It is not difficult to calculate the ease with which it would be to abuse or become addicted to alcohol or illicit substances.

Risk factors are likely to be a major life event, one that induces severe stress. The advent of an unwanted pregnancy which would result in a significant modification of social or employment circumstances might trigger an episode.

It is important that other possible causes for mania are ruled out before making the diagnosis. Certain organic conditions, including cerebral vascular lesions, tumours or certain auto immune diseases may be responsible (Domingues et al. 2016). Illicit stimulant or mood-altering drugs can induce manic symptoms; however, it is clear that any drug induced psychosis, which may present as mania, usually diminishes once the drug is stopped. The use of corticosteroids, antidepressants and thyroid preparations are also associated with manic episodes (Frank et al. 2007).

A lack of sleep or a disturbed sleep pattern can trigger an episode of mania. This can often be the case where night-time child care is shared or where the father is frequently awoken by a crying infant. This is compounded because it may not be a case of insomnia, but more an obsession by the father who believes that he does not require sleep. He needs to remain awake for as long as he is able in order not to waste time any precious time to achieve tasks that could not be done if he were asleep. Consequently, a vicious cycle is created because one of the main components of a manic state is the inability to rest, therefore, the sleep deprivation acts as a catalyst for further mania. There have been claims by Hakkarainen et al. (2003) that the symptoms of bipolar disorder are dictated by seasonal variation, but some studies have refuted this and suggest that there was no evidence to suggest that mania peaked in the lighter summer months whereas depression was more prevalent in the darker, winter months (Murray et al. 2011).

Treatment for acute manic episodes

In severe cases it is pertinent to consider a hospital admission, though it is thought that few fathers would contemplate this, as illustrated in a study by (Fellinger et al. 2018), which found that the number of inpatient episodes was significantly higher in women. However, the average length of stay in both the manic and depressive episode was shorter for women compared to men. The study suggested that despite the equal life time prevalence, severe mood episodes lead to more hospitalisation in women, with men representing one third of all inpatient episodes. This brings into question the efficacy of men to be able to manage their condition or if indeed it is managed at all?

The treatment is antipsychotic medication or valproate for a manic state, with lithium or carbamazepine as the drugs of choice. Clonazepam or lorazepam are recommended for insomnia. Tricyclic antidepressants are often prescribed for depressive symptoms. Sometimes, in severe cases, where the symptoms fail to react to medication and there is a high element of suicidal ideation, electroconvulsive therapy is an option. The effect is often rapid and allows functions to return more quickly.

There are side effects to any psychopharmaceutical treatment and weight gain is one of the more undesirable, and although this is sometimes more pertinent to women, men too are affected by the change in body state and this could be a reason for non-compliance. There is little guarantee that discontinuing medication will result in rapid weight loss. Weight gain also has the debilitating effect of raising blood pressure and increasing cholesterol levels, which bring their own risk factors.

As with all medication, it is advocated that the father be empowered to understand the limitations of the drug, allowing him an element of control on the type of dosage and the time he takes it. If he feels the drugs are over manipulating his mood he may not comply with the quantity and may refuse to take the medication altogether. This will result in a relapse of the condition. It is possible for severe symptoms to endure as long as three months before subsiding, therefore, serum Lithium levels are regularly monitored to ensure the dosage is correct. Compliance with the regime should allow the father to lead a normal, functional life. However, it should be noted that this is a long-term problem with long-term solutions, which requires a modification in lifestyle. Unfortunately, it is not easy for the father to acknowledge the reality of the disorder and denial is often common. This is perhaps due to the fact that the father may find the extreme emotions difficult to deal with (Pipich & Shrand 2018).

Story of a father with bipolar disorder

Storm was studying in university when he was diagnosed with bipolar disorder. He was always a 'jack the lad', frequently getting into trouble with his mates. He was often the ring leader, enticing his mates to play pranks on fellow students. He admitted that often his mates found him 'a bit over the top' and he recognised that he was unaware of his limitations and did not know when to stop his antics. One night, whilst in his hall of residence he felt this surge of energy and found he was unable to sleep, not he said, that he wanted to sleep. In fact, Storm felt so invigorated he turned up his music whilst he danced on his bed. He remembers finally falling into a deep sleep at around 4 am. His mates failed to wake him and he missed lectures. Storm missed many lectures as he now found it almost impossible to get out of bed. He was lethargic, drowsy and neglected to eat. His tutor was made aware of the situation and sent Storm to the occupational health service.

He was sent to the psychiatric services and at twenty years of age was diagnosed with bipolar disorder and put on medication which he managed fairly well and was able to continue in university and gained his degree.

Storm maintained good mental health and took his medication regularly. He met his partner and a year later became a father. Storm couldn't pinpoint why his condition deteriorated but he explained that his sleep pattern was affected and he suffered from insomnia. He stopped his medication, going to the gym and became careless in what he ate, often eating fast food at irregular times. He said he felt overwhelmed with everything, in particular the pressure of being a father. Even though he had a well-paid job, he questioned how he would support his family. He felt terrible doubts about his ability and a creeping feeling about his self-worth and his capability as a father. His confidence was at an all-time low.

Storm started to self-medicate with alcohol and spent longer in the company of his mates. One day he came home and was so euphoric he insisted on slamming the front door and waking the household. His partner was furious, but Storm insisted on rousing his son and sang songs to him whilst dancing him around his nursery. His son cried, his wife cried and ordered him out of the house.

He stayed away for several days and realised he needed to continue with his medication. On his return, however, he avoided being around his son. He said he didn't really feel any love for him but a sense of anger. He told no-one, for fear of the intervention of social services. He 'managed life' until his son was nine months old when Storm felt as if he had hit rock bottom. He had never felt like that. He locked himself in his room, armed with alcohol and had dark thoughts about killing himself. He made the decision to be alone and pushed his whole family away, including his partner. He said that he was hell bent on leaving her and blamed her for wanting a family in the first place. Storm was admitted to a Secure Unit, where he stayed for several weeks. It was there he was able to re-evaluate his situation and get the help he needed to continue with his family life.

Schizophrenia

The exact cause of schizophrenia is unknown, though it has been suggested it may be caused by a combination of physical, psychological, genetic and environmental factors. Having certain infections, though it is unclear what, and being raised in a city, are risk factors. It is thought that poor nutrition during pregnancy can also be a factor (Owen et al. 2016). It is familial, and genetic factors include a variety of common and rare genetic variants. The age of the father also has an influence, as advancing age is a risk factor (Sipos et al. 2004, Luing et al. 2013). Taking cannabis during adolescence heightens the risk of schizophrenia (Kavanagh et al. 2015, Lawrence et al. 2015, Owen et al. 2016).

The prevalence of schizophrenia is about 0.3%–0.7% during a lifetime. Over five years ago there were an estimated 23.6 million cases globally. It appears that men are more often affected and experience more severe symptoms. About a quarter of those suffering make good progress but with fewer recovering completely, as almost half have a lifelong impairment (van Os & Kapur 2009, American Psychiatric Association 2013, Lawrence et al. 2015).

This is often thought of as a split personality but this is a myth; it is a type of psychosis. Recent studies have determined it to be the disturbance of emotions which characterises the illness. The two most common are the termed the 'flattening of affect' and anhedonia. The flattening of affect, usually presents as blunted or diminished expressions of emotion in both the face and the voice. The expression of feelings and emotions are often independent of each other, which means the reaction to a situation is confusing, as sadness may be expressed in a joyous situation. Some have reported the inability to experience pleasure, which is termed anhedonia.

It has been argued that schizophrenia is caused by problems with the neuromotor system, which relates to nerve fibres and impulses passing towards the motor effectors, rather than cognitive deficits. It may be the result of a change in the levels of the neurotransmitters, dopamine and serotonin. The flattening of affect was associated with poorer performance on the right hemisphere of the brain, responsible for comprehension and expression of emotions, relative to the left hemisphere of the brain, which is responsible for expressions of pleasure and anger (Harmon-Jones et al. 2003, Berenbaum et al. 2008a, b).

Two of the important and common symptoms of schizophrenia are delusions and hallucinations. These are considered to be positive symptoms. Delusion is an individual belief or impression which is maintained despite there being evidence to the contrary, either because of the reality of the situation or a rational argument has been stated. Hallucinations are sensory experiences of sight, sound, touch, smell and taste which involve the apparent perception of something which is not present. Hallucinations are thought to be caused because of disturbances in semantic memory and the process of language, whilst delusions are thought to be as a result of cognitive biases (Berenbaum et al. 2008a, b).

There are certain triggers which can precipitate the condition in those who are susceptible to schizophrenia. These include stressful life events such as bereavement, loss of employment or relationship problems. Although a father may not show immediate signs of schizophrenia, facing a stressful episode, such as a traumatic birth or being ill-prepared for the demands of an infant, could generate schizoid reactions, which can cause concern. This can lead to conflict between the parents. Some of the symptoms relating delusions may make it difficult to socialise because of the overwhelming suspicions and distrust.

Concealment of the condition from the public is also a feature and is sometimes a prominent characteristic trait of stigma, as families do not wish to be identified as having a father who is mentally unwell (Phelan et al. 1998, Herbert et al. 2013). However, positive experiences are also prevalent and some have expressed how they felt less selfish and more resilient having a father who suffered from schizophrenia (Herbert et al. 2013). Treatment includes antipsychotic medication and counselling. If there is a serious risk to the father or others then voluntary or involuntary hospitalisation is necessary.

Male postpartum psychosis

There have been a few documented cases of Couvade's Syndrome, also known as 'sympathetic pregnancy' which occurs when the father experiences the same symptoms and behaviours as the expectant mother. This can present as weight gain, nausea, altered hormone levels and sleep disturbances (Trethowan & Conlon 1965). A variety of reasons have been sought for this condition, to include psychosocial and psychoanalytical factors.

The incidence of puerperal psychosis is rare, with an occurrence of two in 1,000 and is most commonly associated with bipolar disorder. Paternal psychosis is even rarer, or rather there are very few reported cases. The florid symptoms tend to present within two to three days following the birth of the infant, but can occur within the next two weeks. The most common symptoms include auditory and visual hallucinations, connected with paranoid and grandiose delusions, which tend to focus around the new-born infant. The intensity of the behaviour and the misconceptions around the infant can jeopardise the safety of both the mother and the infant and therefore prompt treatment is essential (Davenport & Adland 1982, Shapiro & Nass 1986).

However, there was one case reported in 2012 where a father was admitted to a psychiatric unit five days following the birth of his son. The father believed that his son was in danger, and the father was diagnosed with an acute manic episode with psychotic symptoms. The psychological stress he endured precipitated a severe mood disorder. He was successfully treated with hospitalisation, medication and therapy (Shahani 2012).

References

Adler P, Adler P. 2011. Do Men Self-Injure? Male and female patterns of self-harm. *Psychology today on-line* 23rd September. https://www.psychologytoday.com/intl/blog/the-deviance-society/201109/do-men-self-injure, accessed 19 November 2019.

American Psychiatric Association. 2013. *Diagnostic and Statistical Manual of Mental Disorders,* 5th ed. Arlington, VA: Author, pp. 101–105.

Arnold LM. 2003. Gender differences in bipolar disorder. *Psychiatr Clin North Am*, 36(3), pp. 16–25.

Barratt C, Speed W, Green G. 2015. Mental health and houses in multiple occupation. *Journal of Public Mental Health*, 14(2), pp. 107–117.

Baumeister D, Akhtar R, Ciufolini S, Pariante CM, Mondelli V. 2016. Childhood trauma and adult inflammation: A metanalysis of peripheral C-reactive protein, interleukin-6 and tumour necrosis factorα. *Molecular Psychiatry*, 21(5): 642–649.

Berenbaum H, Kerns JG, Vernon LL, Gomez JJ. 2008a. Cognitive correlates of schizophrenia signs and symptoms: II. Emotional disturbances. *Psychiatry Research*, 159(1–2), pp. 157–162.

Berenbaum H, Kerns JG, Vernon LL, Gomez JJ. 2008b. Cognitive correlates of schizophrenia signs and symptoms: III. Hallucinations and delusions. *Psychiatry Research*, 159(1–2), pp. 163–166.

Boyce P, Condon J, Barton J, Corkindale C. 2007. First-Time Fathers' Study: Psychological distress in expectant fathers during pregnancy. *Australian & New Zealand Journal of Psychiatry*, 41, pp. 718–725.

Brennen IR. 2018. Weapon-carrying and the reduction of violent harm. *British Journal of Criminology*, 59(3), pp. 571–593.

Buist A, Morse CA, Durkin S. 2003. Men's adjustment to fatherhood: Implications for obstetric health care. *JOGNN*, 32, pp. 172–180.

Cameron EE, Hunter D, Sedov D, Tomfohr-Madsen M. 2015. What do dads want? Treatment preferences for paternal postpartum depression. *Journal of Affective Disorders*, 215, pp. 62–70.

Dantzer R. 2009. Cytokine, sickness behavior, and depression. *Immunology and Allergy Clinics of North America*, 29, pp. 247–264.

Davenport YB, Adland ML. 1982. Postpartum psychoses in female and male bipolar manic-depressive patients. *American Journal of Orthopsychiatry*, 52, pp. 288–297.

Deater-Deckard K, Pickering K, Dunn JF, Golding J. 1998. Family structure and depressive symptoms in men preceding and following the birth of a child. *American Journal of Psychiatry*, 155, pp. 818–823.

Domingues S, Cotter M, Amado I, Massano R. 2016. Temporal tumor as a cause of bipolarlike disorder? *European Psychiatry*, 41, p. S471.

El-Sayed AM, Haloossim MR, Galea S, Koenen KC. 2012. Epigenetic modifications associated with suicide and common mood and anxiety disorders: A systematic review of the literature. *Biology of Mood & Anxiety Disorders*, 14, p. 10.

Evans GW, Wells NM, Moch A. 2003. Housing and mental health: A review of the evidence and a methodological and conceptual critique. *Journal of Social Issues*, 59(3), pp. 475–500.

Fellinger M, Waldhor T, Bluml V, Nolan W, Vvssoki B. 2018. Influence of gender on inpatient treatment for bipolar disorder: An analysis of 60,607 hospitalisations. *Journal of Affective Disorders*, 225, pp. 104–107.

Fletcher RJ, Matthey S, Marley CG. 2006. Addressing depression and anxiety among new fathers. *MJA*, 185(8), pp. 461–463.

Frank E, Boland E, Novick DM, Bizzarri JV, Rucci P. 2007. Association between illicit drug and alcohol use and first manic episode. *Pharmacology Biochemistry and Behaviour*, 86(2), pp. 395–400.

Goodman JH. 2004. Paternal postpartum depression, its relationship to maternal postpartum depression, and implications for family health. *Journal of Advanced Nursing*, 45(1), pp. 26–35.

Hakkarainen R, Johansson C, Kieseppa T, Partonen T, Koskenvuo M, Jaakko K, Lönnqvist J. 2003. Seasonal changes, sleep length and circadian preference among twins with bipolar disorder. *BMC Psychiatry*, 3, p. 6.

Harmon-Jones E, Sigelman JD, Bohlig A, Harmon-Jones C. 2003. Anger, coping, and frontal cortical activity: The effect of coping potential on anger-induced left frontal activity. *Cognition and Emotion*, 17, pp. 1–24.

Hart BL. 1988. Biological basis of the behavior of sick animals. *Neuroscience & Biobehavioral Reviews*, 12, pp. 123–137.

Hawton K, Saunders KEA, O'Connor R. 2012. Self harm and suicide in adolescents. *Lancet*, 379, pp. 2373–2382.

Herbert HS, Manjula M, Philip M. 2013. Growing up with a parent having schizophrenia: Experiences and resilience in the offspring. *Indian Journal of Psychological Medicine*, 35(2), pp. 148–153.

Holloway T, Gonzalez-Maeso J. 2015. Epigenetic mechanisms of serotonin signaling. *ACS Chemical Neuroscience*, 6(7), pp. 1099–1109.

Johnson MP, Baker SR. 2004. Implications of coping repertoire as predictors of men's stress, anxiety and depression following pregnancy, childbirth and miscarriage: A longitudinal study. *Journal of Psychosomatic Obstetrics and Gynecology*, 25, pp. 87–98.

Kavanagh DH, Tansey KE, O'Donovan MC, Owen MJ. 2015. Schizophrenia genetics: Emerging themes for a complex disorder. *Molecular Psychiatry*, 20(1), pp. 72–76.

Kerr DCR, Owen LD, Capaldi DM. 2008. Suicidal ideation and its recurrence in boys and men from early adolescence to early adulthood: An event analysis. *Journal of Abnormal Psychology*, 117, pp. 625–636.

Klonsky D, Muehlenkamp J. 2007. Self-injury: A research review for the practitioner. *Journal of Clinical Psychology: In Session*, 63(11), pp. 1045–1056.

Kopeykina I, Kim HJ, Khatun T, Boland J, Haeri S, Cohen LJ, Galynker II. 2016. Hypersexuality and couple relationships in bipolar disorder: A review. *Journal of Affective Disorders*, 195, pp. 1–14.

Lawrence RE, First MB, Lieberman JA. 2015. Chapter 48: Schizophrenia and other psychoses. In: Tasman A, Kay J, Lieberman JA, First MB, Riba MB. (Eds), *Psychiatry*, 4th ed. Chichester: John Wiley & Sons, Ltd, pp. 791–856.

Luing T, Lichtenstein P, Sandin S, Hultman C, D'Onofrio BM, Langstom N, Larsson H. 2013. The association between parental schizophrenia and offspring suicide: A cousin comparison approach. *Psychological Medicine*, 43(3), pp. 581–590.

Maes M, Berk M, Goehler L, Song C, Anderson G, Gałecki P, Leonard B. 2012. Depression and sickness behavior are Janus-faced responses to shared inflammatory pathways. *BMC Med*, 10, p. 66.

Matthey S, Barnett B, Ungerer J, Waters B. 2000. Paternal and maternal depressed mood during the transition to parenthood. *Journal of Affective Disorders*, 60, pp. 75–85.

Murray G, Lam R, Beaulieu S, Sharma V, Cervantes P, Parikh SV, Yatham LN. 2011. Do symptoms of bipolar disorder exhibit seasonal variation? A multi prospective investigation. *Bipolar Disorders*, 13(7–8), pp. 687–695.

ONS Office for National Statistics. 2018. Suicides in the UK 2017 registrations. https://www.ons.gov.uk/peoplepopulationandcommunity/birthsdeathsandmarriages/deaths/bulletins/suicidesintheunitedkingdom/2017registrations, accessed 19 November 2019.

ONS Office for National Statistics. 2015. Suicides in the UK 2013. https://www.ons.gov.uk/peoplepopulationandcommunity/birthsdeathsandmarriages/deaths/bulletins/suicidesintheunitedkingdom/2015-02-19, accessed 19 November 2019.

van Os J, Kapur S. 2009. Schizophrenia. *Lancet*, 374(9690), pp. 635–45.

Owen MJ, Sawa A, Mortensen PB. 2016. Schizophrenia. *Lancet*, 388(10039), pp. 86–97.

Paulson JF, Bazemore SD. 2010. Prenatal and postpartum depression in fathers and its association with maternal depression: A meta-analysis. *JAMA*, 303(19), pp. 1961–1969.

Phelan JC, Bromet EJ, Link BG. 1998. Psychiatric illness and family stigma. *Schizophr Bull*, 24, pp. 115–126.

Pitt B. 1993. *Down with Gloom*. London: Gaskell Press and Royal College of Psychiatrists.

Pipich M, Shrand J. 2018. *Owning Bipolar: How Patients and Families Can Take Control of Bipolar Disorder*. New York: Citadel Press.

Quevedo L, da Silva RA, Coelho F, Pinheiro KA, Horta BL, Kapczinski F, Pinheiro RT. 2011. Risk of suicide and mixed episode in men in the postpartum period. *Journal of Affective Disorders*, 132(1–2), pp. 243–246.

Saxbe DE, Schetter CD, Simon CD, Adam EK, Shalowitz MU. High. 2017. Paternal testosterone may protect against postpartum depressive symptoms in fathers, but confer risk to mothers and children. *Hormones and Behavior*, 95, p. 103.

Schmaal L, Veltman D, van Erp TG et al. 2015. Subcortical brain alterations in major depressive disorder: Findings from the ENIGMA Major Depressive Disorder working group. *Molecular Psychiatry*, 21(6), pp. 806–812.

Schumacher M, Zubaran C, White G. 2008. Bringing birth-related paternal depression to the fore. *Women Birth*, 21(2), pp. 65–70.

Shahani L. 2012. A father with postpartum psychosis. *BMJ Case Reports*, doi: 10.1136/bcr.11.2011.5176.

Shapiro S, Nass J. 1986. Postpartum psychosis in the male. *Psychopathology*, 19, p. 138.

Sipos A, Rasmussen F, Harrison G, Leon DA, Gunnell D. 2004. Paternal age and schizophrenia: A population-based cohort study. *BMJ*, 329(7474), p. 1070.

Sun BQ, Zhang J. 2016. Economic and sociological correlates of suicides: Multilevel analysis of the time series data in the United Kingdom. *Journal of Forensic Sciences*, 61(2), pp. 345–351.

Trethowan WH, Conlon MF. 1965. The Couvade syndrome. *The British Journal of Psychiatry*, 111(470), pp. 57–66.

World Health Organisation. 2016. *Mental Health Suicide Statistics*. Geneva: WHO Press.

Young S. 2007. How to increase serotonin in the human brain without drugs. *Journal of Psychiatry & Neuroscience*, 32(6), pp. 394–399.

Chapter 5

Cross cutting themes

The cross-cutting themes of eating disorders and substance misuse can apply to any mental disorder or illness. The stigma of mental illness and shame sometimes forces fathers to seek to self-medicate in order to improve their mental status. In some cases, fathers may feel they are succeeding but are ignorant of the fact that they are actually causing more damage.

Eating disorders

Approximately 10% of people with eating disorders are men. Some articles have suggested that during their lifetime 0.3% of men will experience anorexia, 0.5% will experience bulimia and 2% will experience binge eating disorder. Men make up 40% of people diagnosed with binge eating disorder (Hudson et al. 2007, Eisenberg et al. 2012). More men appear to have bulimia rather than anorexia, with the prevalence increasing over the past fifteen years. The National Centre for Mental Health (2018) suggests that over one and half a million people in the UK have an eating disorder.

The difference between men and women are their weight histories as men were usually mild to moderately obese, prior to developing an eating disorder, particularly if they were obese during childhood. Conversely, women typically, had a normal weight history (Storther et al. 2012).

There are three classifications applied to eating disorders. Anorexia is characterised by low bodyweight primarily caused by the restriction of food in order to avoid weight gain. Bulimia nervosa is characterised by binge eating and then voiding, either by vomiting or taking laxatives, to avoid any further weight gain. Binge eating has no restricting behaviours, which results in obesity because of the amount of food consumed (Weltzin 2005). The eating disorders of anorexia and bulimia are usually centred around controlling the amount of nutrients consumed. In severe cases these may be limited sufficiently to maintain life, or in less severe cases to control the body size. A combination of measures may be used to ensure weight is maintained. These can include purging by inducing vomiting following a large meal or taking laxatives to guarantee frequent bowel movements. Fasting is one way to be certain that there is no gain in weight.

Eating disorders are usually associated with anxiety, depression and substance misuse and the potential risk factors appear be previous criticism about eating habits from a teacher, parent or sibling. The reasons for eating disorders are complex and multifactorial. There does not appear to be a single risk factor but a combination of genetics, psychological, physiological, social and environmental issues, though there is a school of thought that suggests eating disorders are more biologically based than was previously thought.

Anorexia

Anorexia usually develops in adolescence and lasts for approximately six years. Anorexia was once primarily a condition suffered by girls, but in recent years there has been an increasing number of boys. Low bodyweight has a significant impact on lifestyle and in the worst-case scenario may result in death. The problem is that anorexia changes the body's physiology and lowers testosterone levels. Treatment of the disorder, and the subsequent weight gain, can reverse the process and reinstate puberty (Pritchard 2008). However, although difficult to treat, over half of those who have the condition will fully recover.

Bulimia

Bulimia is less likely in men as they tend to avoid vomiting and laxatives (Morgan 2008). Women tend to get angry with themselves because they have succumbed to overeating, but men tend to binge or over indulge, because they are angry. It is not easy to diagnose because the alterations in body mass are difficult to detect and the restricting behaviours are often concealed. Binge eating disorder involves eating large quantities of food over a short period of time. It is difficult to stop and often the fathers feel disconnected from the food and have difficulty remembering what they have eaten. It is usually ritualistic whereby particular foods are purchased in order to consume large amounts, or it can be spontaneous when the opportunity arises. Whatever the reasons, the father is generally overwhelmed by guilt and disgust at his inability to stop this behaviour, but this is not as overstated as it is with women.

Primarily the father may be suffering from body dysmorphia where there is an unrealistic belief in their actual body size. The populist emphasis is that men's bodies should be toned and muscular. This is depicted within the media arena, portraying the man with the 'six pack' chest being the more desirable. Magazines and adverts subscribe to the process of maintaining bodyweight by accentuating the plethora of dietary products which are available to help tone and develop a powerful body structure. It is thought that a significant number of teenage boys partake in extreme exercise, usually in the gym, with the direct object of bulking up their bodies, as this is a more acceptable form of behaviour (Storther et al. 2012).

However, men suffering from eating disorders are usually less likely to seek help, because they may not recognise their obsession with body image as being a problem, as this condition relates mainly to women. Their reluctance to access support is reiterated by the stigma of mental illness and the reaction they think they will encounter. The attitude surrounding weight gain is probably one of the most robust types of stigma (Puhl et al. 2009); therefore, the pressure to conform is probably stronger in the man who views his body as grossly overweight. It would, however, appear that men are becoming more aware of the implications of the disorder and are seeking help.

Participating in a programme that is predominately tailored for females may also be a barrier. Although there is emerging research into eating disorders in mothers during the perinatal period by Easter et al. (2013), there is little research into the effect this has on fathers and their capabilities in parenthood. However, with the emphasis primarily on women's treatment options, a more male focussed approach might be more appropriate.

As with all eating disorders, the illness is not about the consumption of food but the feelings the father is experiencing. The way in which they interact with food and the rituals surrounding eating sometimes helps to cope with anxiety and or depressive symptoms. However, it has been suggested that too often, the father's body shape has to have changed significantly before it is recognised that he has an eating disorder, which is why campaigners like Virgo (2019) are insisting that attitudes need to change and realise it is about the emotions rather than food.

Story of a father with an eating disorder

Bryn's story: *I honestly can't remember when I started vomiting and over using laxatives but certainly went in overdrive when things happened in my family.*

I had always used the gym for at least three hours a day. I was obsessed with looking good but deep down I knew I was suffering with real anxiety before I became a parent. I learnt to escape and hide my feelings and actions from my wife.

When my daughter was born, it changed our relationship. My wife had to return to work, I had to care for my daughter. I wasn't able to get to the gym after work, so instead I took the baby out in the pram and walked for hours on end and counted the calories that way. I became obsessed with taking my daughter out in the pram, even in the colder weather. This caused rows and my eating habits changed far worse.

I'd increase my amount of times I made myself vomit. That meant my teeth were getting worse and was suffering from bad breath. I started to feel paranoid about my body shape and stopped going out and started doing exercises in the house.

I downloaded an app which helped to count the calories and became obsessed with that, checking my phone every time I ate something. I thought it was really useful. It allowed me to record everything I ate, even if it was a grape. If the app said I wasn't eating enough, that was great as it meant

I was actually beating the app. If I could radically cut what I was eating then I felt really good about myself. It was like a badge of honour! I could actually survive on fewer calories than I was supposed to! So, that was great. I was also going onto chat forums to find out other ways in which I could lose my weight and tone up my body. I was on my mobile so often I realised I preferred to look at what was on my screen than look at my daughter. If I am honest, I got irritated if she distracted me. I realised though, that I was really starting to neglect my daughter.

I was never diagnosed by the clinicians and only went to see the doctor when I felt poorly and found that my blood pressure was high. I was feeling anger and my marriage was in pieces. I don't even know why I started smoking to stop the craving of food.

One thing I do know I went for counselling after my partner wanted me to leave and told her everything, even about my childhood trauma and not being connected to my parents. I received intense CBT and had online support. I do now exercise but only to keep healthy. After months of getting better I don't want my daughter seeing me and copying my actions either.

Self-medication and substance misuse

Depressive symptoms, the experiences and perceptions, are some of the risk factors which are associated with substance misuse and with them comes an increased risk of poorer outcomes when treating the depression. Evidence suggests that there is a greater likelihood of substance misuse when depression is present.

The habit is a two-way process, as abuse of substances is more likely to cause and intensify depression whilst those who suffer from depression are more likely to abuse substances. The reasons are clear as sometimes, the intolerable symptoms of despair and guilt are temporarily relieved; however, most of the substances can have a depressive effect and increase the feelings of sadness and fatigue. This is sometimes the case with those who have bipolar disorder who appear to benefit from the same perceived advantages of elevating their depression and calming their mania. Chronic abuse can unmask bipolar disorder and cause an increase in the severity of the symptoms.

The greater the symptoms of depression the more the belief that substance misuse has social benefits, as there tends to be higher levels of this practice amongst peers and friends (Siennick et al. 2017). Initially the substances may minimise or moderate the symptoms, but when withdrawal is attempted following chronic abuse, this exacerbates the depressive feelings and leads to an increase in abuse and ultimately dependence. Abstinence, however, brings its own difficulties, as taking the substance masks the feelings and when this is no longer the case, these symptoms reappear, with equal vigour. A combination of these symptoms makes treatment problematic.

Caffeine abuse

Caffeine abuse is the most commonly used drug with over 90% of adults using it regularly. The average consumption is two cups of coffee a day or five cans of soft drink (Higdon & Frei 2006). Low doses of the drug are relatively safe, but when the consumption is greater this leads to physical and mental ill health. It is possible to become dependent upon or addicted to caffeine and despite the obvious health risks, some find it difficult to reduce their intake (Anderson & Juliano 2012).

Caffeine in the form of coffee is very palatable, and with the advent of commercial coffee houses, increases the opportunity for social gatherings in towns and communities. Drinking copious cups of coffee seems to be one of the more acceptable substance misuses. As it is a stimulant, it can increase energy levels, alertness and overall wellbeing, and it is possible to tolerate high doses. However, the adverse reaction is the physical effects of disruptive sleep and problems with hypertension. For fathers who are working or studying there are many excuses for consuming coffee, primarily because of the need to stay awake, alert and to aid concentration. The father may notice that if he tries to cut down or stop, he can suffer from debilitating headaches and cravings (Meredith et al. 2013). A glass of water could be a substation for a cup of coffee, but this may also be met with derision or contempt. However, the knowledge that they are harming their mental state might persuade the father to rethink his stimulation habits. A slow introduction over a two-week period may seem more acceptable.

The indications of caffeine abuse may include restlessness, agitation, verbosity, insomnia, gastrointestinal and cardiac disturbances and diuresis, allowing for the fact that these conditions do not have an organic cause. The dependency on caffeine has been categorised into a mild, moderate or severe disorder. The criteria include, that despite knowing the risks, there is a craving for large amounts of caffeine, there has been an attempt to reduce and control the intake and there are characteristic signs of caffeine withdrawal (DSM5 2013). The signs of caffeine tolerance are defined by a marked increase in the amount of caffeine consumed in order to achieve the desired effect, often because the existing amount is insufficient. There is also a noticeable amount of time spent in activities designed to obtain, use or recover from the effects of caffeine (DSM5 2013).

There is increasing evidence to suggest that dependence on caffeine is a clinical disorder (WHO 2018, DSM 5th edition). Caffeine acts as an antagonist at adenosine receptors, blocking endogenous adenosine (Daly 1993). It produces a range of behavioural stimulant effects and one study suggested that paraxanthine, which is the primary metabolite in caffeine, produces an increase in locomotor activity (Orru et al. 2013). There is a neurochemical mechanism which underlies the withdrawal. When there is abstinence from caffeine there is increased functional sensitivity to adenosine which plays an important role in the behavioural and physiological effect.

There is an increasing preference for sugary, soft drinks and energy drinks which contain high levels of caffeine. This allows more caffeine to be consumed in smaller portions, sometimes resulting in caffeine intoxication. This can cause both physical and mental health problems and rarely, death (Juliano et al. 2011).

There is little research on the comorbidity of caffeine and another drug dependency. Some have shown that those addicted to caffeine were also more likely to be dependent on cigarette smoking and alcohol abuse. A common genetic factor on polysubstance use has been postulated, but this area requires further research (Hughes et al. 2000, Kendler et al. 2007, Striley et al. 2011).

Cocaine and amphetamines

Cocaine and amphetamines are stimulants which are often easily accessible and are used by some fathers to exhilarate and energise in order to annihilate any morbid feelings they have. For some fathers, drug taking is becoming ingrained within their social circles. The drugs alter the serotonin transporter that causes dysfunction within the neural reward pathways. Chronic use of these may produce symptoms typical of bipolar disorder to include increased energy, hypomania, paranoia and grandiose ideation. When attempts are made to withdraw from the drug, it can produce the reverse symptoms of apathy, hopelessness and, in some cases, cause suicidal ideation.

Alcohol

In England 26% of men drank alcohol above the safe recommended limits. Almost 9% were alcohol dependent and 7.8% showed mild dependence (ONS 2014). Alcohol alters the levels of serotonin and its metabolites to lower than normal levels. This increases sensitivity, which contributes to the progression from the occasional use of alcohol to the more intense, habitual addiction. Intoxication can produce symptoms of mania.

The most common excuse for drinking alcohol is that it reduces feelings of stress and improves the mood. A visit to the pub on the way home from a stressful day at the office is twofold as the father has the experience of socialising with company who have similar interests and the pleasure of an intoxicating substance. Alternatively, there is the quiet drink of supermarket whiskey whilst on the PlayStation. The immediate effect of the alcohol placates the mind. It has been suggested that alcohol is often used to manage depressive symptoms because it offers a quick fix and feelings of sadness can briefly dissipate (Young-Wolff et al. 2009, Boden & Fergusson 2011).

There are several reasons why alcohol consumption and mood disorders may be linked. One explanation is the abuse of alcohol can exacerbate already dysfunctional relationships and social circumstances (Fergusson et al. 2009). A genetic link has been suggested, relating to the functioning of the neurotransmitters, which increase the risk of depression when alcohol has been consumed. There has been evidence of increased risks of both depression and alcohol abuse with those who have a particular genotype. Studies have found that particular variants of the eleven muscarinic acetylcholine receptor M2 gene are related to increased risks to both alcoholism and depression (Wang et al. 2004, Luo et al. 2005, Kuo et al. 2010). There is a suggestion that alcohol abuse causes metabolic changes that increase the risk of depression. Reduced folate levels have been linked to risks of depression (Mceachin et al. 2008).

It is advised to make a clinical assessment only following a reasonable period of abstinence. This allows the symptoms of acute intoxication and withdrawal symptoms to subside. Studies have found there was a significant decrease in depressive symptoms from the first day of abstinence to the end of the second week (Goldsmith & Ries 2003, Quello et al. 2005). The recovery rate from alcohol tends to be shorter than that of the amphetamines or cocaine, which may require several weeks. During this period support and supervision are necessary, which may mean hospitalisation or significant input from a crisis team. The presentation of the more severe withdrawal symptoms may require immediate treatment rather than waiting for the time to elapse.

Discussing the substitution of beer with a non-alcoholic variety may be met with derision, whilst currently the flavours and impact are unsatisfactory. However, non-alcoholic ciders are much improved and could easily be substituted if the father has a desire to try to change his lifestyle.

There is an association between substance misuse, depression and suicide, with the disinhibition and despair linked to intoxication. This carries a high risk which can lead to impulsive and self-destructive acts.

Analgesics and opioid misuse

The use of opioids appears to be increasing and, as with the linkage with other substances and mood disorders, it is bi-directional. The misuse of opiates is defined when they are used for non-medical reasons or when a greater dosage is consumed than has been prescribed. They can, however, conceal as well as elevate the symptoms of depression and it has been noted that opiates are less effective if depression is already present. If the father presents with back pain or headache, rather than a diagnosis of depression, it is probable that opioids will be the treatment of choice. Some fathers with depression may overuse the opioids because they find the mellowing effects more helpful for treating their insomnia and stress. This compensates for the reduced endogenous opioid response to stressors. If depression is present, it has been found that some will continue to use opioids even when the pain is less severe. Studies have shown that long-term opioid use increases the risk of the incidence, recurrence and treatment-resistant depression (Murphy et al. 2018a, b, Sullivan 2018).

The abuse can be determined by the consideration of the habit of taking the opioids. Some of the signs of opioid abuse include the father sleeping at odd hours, being constantly tired or down, with frequent mood changes, which alter from being pleasant to being unusually irritable and agitated. Unsuccessfully attempting to reduce the dosage, because the cravings are overwhelming, exacerbates the problem. The amount of time spent acquiring and recovering from the effects of the drug is also a sign of over usage, particularly if it interferes with the father's work and recreational pursuits. The potent effects of the drug can sometimes cause difficulties within relationships, but the desire for the drug is so consuming it negates the need to discontinue it.

As with other addictions the most promising type of treatment is talking and behavioural therapies coupled with antidepressants. The addition of the drug methadone or naltrexone can help to treat the dependence on the opioid.

Heroin is sometimes the drug of choice because painkillers are no longer affective. This is one of the strongest opiates and appears to be more readily available and, in some cases, cheaper than ordinary opiates. Heroin addiction can mimic the signs of depression and lead to anhedonia and despair. Heroin users are at increased risk of suicide. The withdrawal symptoms can be severe and include nausea, vomiting, stomach cramps, sweating and disrupted sleep all of which require medical as well as psychological attention.

However, tailored programmes which reduce the cravings and concentrate on depressive symptoms can improve the recovery. One study found there was no consistent evidence for treating substance misuse, except the suggestion that those without substance misuse had a greater increase in psychotherapy (Watkins et al. 2006). Antidepressants are usually prescribed for both substance misuse and the depression. The more effective treatment is a combination of talking and behavioural therapies. In some cases, admission to an inpatient facility is often the best recourse as substance abstinence, and subsequently withdrawal can be managed in tandem with learning and implementing coping strategies for the depression.

Cognitive-behavioural therapies (CBTs) are found to be amongst the most effective psychosocial treatments. Those addicted to alcohol, when treated, had a greater improvement in their depressive symptoms and better drinking outcomes (Weiss et al. 2000).

The abuse of substances, however, has an adverse effect on the process and prognosis of mood disorders, which leads to treatment resistant programmes. However, alleviation in the symptoms which present can improve the substance related outcomes (Siennick et al. 2017).

Story of a father with substance misuse

Ben had been diagnosed with personality disorder. He had followed his older brother in the gang culture after their father left the family home after years of abuse. His younger brother lived at home with his mother who suffered from postnatal depression. Ben started abusing drugs, particularly amphetamines (speed), at the age of twelve and although he experimented with various drugs, his preference was for speed. He managed to work in the local factory but was only on the minimum wage. Ben had always suffered from low self esteem, and always thought he was not as good or as clever as his peers. He did not feel he fitted in anywhere, and seemed to have lost all purpose.

Ben did not have any real ambitions in life and his lifestyle was chaotic. He was used to disorder and confusion in his world. When he was twenty-seven years of age, Ben and Ell met and this relationship started to change his pattern of behaviours. He became less reliant on drugs but still used them when he needed a quick fix. However, when Ben became a father, he made the decision to give up the drug habit. He did not want to be the bad father his father was, but he needed help to stop taking speed. He made the decision to sign up for the gym as he felt that would help him take his mind off his mood. Ben decided to take a keen interest in the antenatal classes to prepare himself for fatherhood. He even sought out cognitive behavioural therapy and because he was so impressed with the help it gave him, Ben decided he would take on a therapist course to help others like himself. Ben is now a successful therapist and a successful father.

Cannabis

Cannabis is the most widely used recreational drug in the world. It is a combination of stems, leaves and flower buds of the cannabis sativa plant. It can be smoked, eaten or vaporised. When smoked, it is spread onto rolling papers and formed into a cigarette, called a joint. Smoking releases the tetrahydrocannabinol (THC), contained in the cannabis, which is absorbed into the lungs and through the blood stream. It can be ingested by adding to foodstuffs. It can be brewed as a tea or added to milk or soft drinks. Vaporising is done using the same system as e-cigarettes. Tetrahydrocannabinol is responsible for the feelings of euphoria. During the past forty years the potency of TCH content has risen to over 30%, which makes it difficult to determine the short- and long-term effects of cannabis.

Over thirty years ago the link was made between cannabis use and the risk of psychosis. However, it was not established whether the use was caused by a pre-existing psychosis rather than the result of taking the drug. Using cannabis in adolescence does increase the possibility of experiencing psychotic symptoms in adulthood. Most, however, are unharmed by using cannabis, and some fathers will admit to using it to calm their nerves or to find some inner peace in their turbulent world. However, its use should be avoided in those who are particularly psychologically vulnerable (Andréasson et al. 1987, Arseneault et al. 2002).

Cannabis use is approximately 2.5 times more common amongst those with anxiety and depression (RCP & RCPsych 2013). One study found an association with risk of developing depression and suicidal behaviour in later life, however, there was no association with anxiety. The risk to the father, in itself is moderate to low, but the suggestion that the high number of adolescents who currently consume cannabis now indicates the large number who may develop depression and suicide ideation later in life, and that of course, can include fathers (Gobbi et al. 2019).

The ingestion of cannabis, similar to alcohol and tobacco, affects the sperm count and its vitality. One study found high concentrations in the urine, which corresponded to a lower sperm count and changes in the genetic profiling, however, it was unable to determine if this affected fertilisation or the future health of their offspring (Murphy et al. 2018a, b). The changes in the quantity and the quality of the sperm might not be permanent as new sperm is generated daily and takes about ten weeks to mature. If not ejaculated the sperm die and are reabsorbed back into the body. Therefore, in the absence of cannabis, new sperm can develop normally. In light of this research, it is probably advisable to cease taking cannabis at least six months prior to conceiving (Murphy et al. 2018a, b).

Smoking tobacco

In the UK of the ten million people smoke, almost one in three have mental health problems. Those who suffer from a major depressive disorder were more likely to smoke on a regular basis than those with no psychiatric history, and are also less likely to be able to stop the habit (Glassman et al. 1990). This prevalence has not changed over the past twenty years. Evidence suggests that when smoking is stopped, the symptoms of depression return. There are seven withdrawal symptoms listed in the DSM3 (1986), but depression is not one of them.

The association between smoking and mental disorders is complex. Smoking tends to be higher in those fathers who are alcohol or drug dependent. Almost half of adults in England who are dependent on alcohol and 69% of those who take drugs, are smokers, and there is the risk that fathers who smoke are more likely to smoke cannabis (Gfroerer et al. 2002). Smoking is more hazardous to the health of those being treated for substance misuse than the actual substance. If smoking is continued, it appears to hamper the process of cognitive recovery after there is also abstinence from alcohol (Kalman et al. 2010). Those fathers who are treated with benzodiazepines and opiates, require higher doses of the drug, because of the induction of liver enzymes by tobacco smoke (Carrillo et al. 2003).

The inhalation of nicotine damages the pathways in the amygdala and may trigger mood swings and, in particular, the inhibition of negative emotions. It alters the balance of both dopamine and noradrenaline. The initial rush of euphoria is produced by the surge of nicotine, and it has been suggested that whilst higher doses act as a stimulant, low doses can have a depressant effect. The changes occur rapidly, which is why it can produce dependency as more smoking occurs: the more the brain becomes addicted to, and the need for, a feeling of euphoria. Smoking appears to ameliorate the symptoms of anxiety whilst nicotine withdrawal exacerbates the symptoms of anxiety and depression.

It has been found that taking antidepressant medication can prevent recurrence of the symptoms, particularly stress and anxiety. These are exacerbated by the physical symptoms of breathlessness and headaches, and it is for that reason that many decide they need to continue smoking. Gaining weight, through stopping smoking, which is exacerbated by low levels of exercise and the effect of some medication, proves a significant problem. There can be a weight gain of over 5 kg (Fontaine et al. 2001, Lycett et al. 2011).

There are several smoking cessation programmes, and it has been proven that quitting smoking is more likely to happen if there is support and monitoring for the father. The complexities of reducing the number of cigarettes smoked are multiple and can create challenges with not only motivation, but having the confidence to completely stop. Harm reduction can offer potential benefits and the notion of reducing the intake with a view to eventually stopping is for some, a more acceptable strategy.

Story of a father who smoked

Mo had smoked since he was a teenager and whenever he felt stressed, he would reach out for the packet of cigarettes. He had always been told by his group of friends that smoking would help calm him down.

When Mo's partner became pregnant, he realised that money was going to be tight, and he could not really afford the price of cigarettes and be able to buy for his new baby. His partner had been advised by the midwife that she should give up smoking as it would be detrimental to the baby's health, but there was no mention of Mo being asked to give it up. Mo, however, was anxious that both he and his partner gave up smoking but it was increasingly difficult as neither could manage to stop at the same time. The realisation, however, of the importance of a smoke-free pregnancy and the possibility of bringing a baby into a smoke-filled home, gave them the impetus they needed to stop.

During the antenatal class they took note of the smoking cessation classes and made a determined effort to stop. It was not easy and there were times when Mo became very irritated with his partner and vice versa. Mo said, 'I felt I had to do the best for my boy. I did not want him to have a mum and dad that were constantly smoking, or us dying with lung cancer while he was still young. It was hard but we did it. My stress is less too as I learnt new stuff in the relaxation classes, and my mate showed me a mindfulness app to help to give me focus when I am feeling overwhelmed or stressed'.

Each of the themes is synonymous of typical male pursuits. Most of the substances are easily acquired and negate the need to visit a doctor or consult a health professional. The habit can seriously compromise any diagnosis or treatment and also inhibits further research into why fathers feel forced to initiate these behaviours and why they are so compulsive and addictive.

References

American Psychiatric Association, 1986. *Diagnostic and Statistical Manual of Mental Disorders*, 3rd ed. Washington DC: Author.

American Psychiatric Association, 2013. *Diagnostic and Statistical Manual of Mental Disorders*, 5th ed. Arlington VA: Author.

Anderson BL, Juliano LM. 2012. Behavior, sleep, and problematic caffeine consumption in a college-aged sample. *Journal Caffeine Research*, 2, pp. 38–44.

Andréasson S, Allebeck P, Engström A, Rydberg U. 1987. Cannabis and schizophrenia: A longitudinal study of Swedish conscripts. *Lancet*, 2(8574), pp. 1483–1485.

Arseneault L, Cannon M, Poulton R, Murray R, Caspi A, Moffitt TE. 2002. Cannabis use in adolescence and risk for adult psychosis: Longitudinal prospective study. *British Medical Journal (Clinical Research Ed.)*, 325(7374), pp. 1212–1213.

Boden JM, Fergusson DM. 2011. Alcohol and depression. *Addiction*, 106, pp. 906–914.

Carrillo JA, Herraiz AG, Ramos SI et al. 2003. Role of the smoking-induced cytochrome P450 (CYP)1A2 and polymorphic CYP2D6 in steady-state concentration of olanzapine. *Journal of Clinical Psychopharmacology*, 23(2), pp. 119–127.

Daly JW. 1993. Mechanism of action of caffeine. In: Garattini S (Ed.), *Caffeine, Coffee, and Health*. New York: Raven Press, pp. 97–150.

Easter A, Taborelli E, Corfield F, Schmidt U, Treasure J, Micali N. 2013. Recognising the symptoms: How common are eating disorders in pregnancy? *European Eating Disorders Review*, 21(4), pp. 340–344.

Eisenberg M, Wall M, Neumark-Sztainer D. 2012. Muscle-enhancing behaviors among adolescent girls and boys. *Pediatrics* 130(6), pp. 1019–1026.

Fergusson DM, Boden JM, Horwood LJ. 2009. Tests of causal links between alcohol abuse or dependence and major depression. *Archive of General Psychiatry*, 66, pp. 260–266.

Fontaine KR, Heo M, Harrigan EP et al. 2001. Estimating the consequences of antipsychotic induced weight gain on health and mortality rate. *Psychiatry Research*, 101, pp. 277–288.

Gfroerer JC, Wu LT, Penne MA. 2002. *Initiation of Marijuana Use: Trends, Patterns, and Implications* (Analytic Series: A-17, DHHS Publication No. SMA 02-3711). Rockville, MD: Substance Abuse and Mental Health Services Administration, Office of Applied Studies.

Glassman AH, Helzer JE, Covey LS, Cottler LB, Stetner F, Tipp JE, Johnson J. 1990. Smoking, smoking cessation, and major depression. *Journal of the American Medical Association*, 264, pp. 1546–1549.

Gobbi G, Atkin T, Zytynski T et al. 2019. Association of cannabis use in adolescence and risk of depression, anxiety, and suicidality in young adulthood. A systematic review and meta-analysis. *Journal of the American Medical Association Psychiatry*, 76(4), pp. 426–434. doi: 10.1001/jamapsychiatry.2018.4500.

Goldsmith RJ, Ries RK. 2003. Substance-induced mental disorders. In: Graham AW, Schultz TK, Mayo-Smith MF, Ries RK, Wilford BB (Eds), *Principles of Addiction Medicine*, 3rd ed. Maryland: Chevy Chase, pp. 1263–1276.

Higdon JV, Frei B. 2006. Coffee and health: A review of recent human research. *Critical Reviews in Food Science Nutrition*, 46(2), pp. 101–123.

Hudson JI, Hiripi E, Pope HG Jr, Kessler RC. 2007. The prevalence and correlates of eating disorders in the national comorbidity survey replication. *Biological Psychiatry*, 161(3), pp. 348–358.

Hughes JR, Oliveto AH, MacLaughlin M. 2000. Is dependence on one drug associated with dependence on other drugs? The cases of alcohol, caffeine and nicotine. *American Journal on Addictions*, 9(3), pp. 196–201.

Juliano LM, Anderson BL, Griffiths RR. 2011. Caffeine. In: Ruiz P, Strain E (Eds), *Lowinson & Ruiz's Substance Abuse: A Comprehensive Textbook*. 5th ed. Philadelphia: Lippincott Williams & Wilkins, pp. 335–353.

Kalman D, Kim S, DiGirolamo G, Smelson D, Ziedonis D. 2010. Addressing tobacco use disorder in smokers in early remission from alcohol dependence: The case for integrating smoking cessation services in substance use disorder treatment programs. *Clinical Psychology Review*, 30(1), pp. 12–24.

Kendler KS, Myers J, Prescott CA. 2007. Specificity of genetic and environmental risk factors for symptoms of cannabis, cocaine, alcohol, caffeine, and nicotine dependence. *Archives of General Psychiatry*, 64(11), pp. 1313–1320.

Kuo PH, Neale MC, Walsh D et al. 2010. Genome-wide linkage scans for major depression in individuals with alcohol dependence. *Journal of Psychiatric Research*, 44(9), pp. 616–619.

Luo X, Kranzler HR, Zuo L et al. 2005. CHRM2 gene predisposes to alcohol dependence, drug dependence and affective disorders: Results from an extended case-control structured association study. *Human Molecular Genetics*, 14, pp. 2421–2434.

Lycett D, Murphy M, Aveyard P. 2011. Associations between weight change over 8 years and baseline body mass index in a cohort of continuing and quitting smokers. *Addiction*, 106, pp. 188–196.

Mceachin RC, Keller BJ, Saunders EF, Mcinnis MG. 2008. Modeling gene-by-environment interaction in comorbid depression with alcohol use disorders via an integrated bioinformatics approach. *BioData Mining*, 1, p. 2.

Meredith SE, Juliano LM, Hughes JR, Griffiths RR. 2013. Caffeine use disorder: A comprehensive review and research agenda. *Journal of Caffeine Research*, 3(3), pp. 114–130.

Morgan J. 2008. *The Invisible Man: A Self-Help Guide for Men with Eating Disorders, Compulsive Exercise, and Bigorexia*. New York, NY: Routledge.

Murphy DL, Lebin JA, Severtson SG, Olsen HA, Dasgupta N, Dart RC. 2018a. Comparative rates of mortality and serious adverse effects among commonly prescribed opioid analgesics. *Drug Safety*, 41(8), pp. 787–795.

Murphy SK, Itchon-Ramos N, Visco Z, Huang C, Grenier R, Schott K. et al. 2018b. Cannabinoid exposure and altered DNA methylation in rat and human sperm. *Journal of Epigenetics*, 13(12), pp. 1208–1221.

National Centre for Mental Health. 2018. Eating disorder statistics. https://www.ncmh.info › 2018/04/30 › battling-anorexia, accessed 19 November 2019.

Office for National Statistics. 2014. Adult Psychiatric Morbidity Survey: Survey of Mental Health and Wellbeing, England 1993–2014. https://digital.nhs.uk/data-and-information/publications/statistical/adult-psychiatric-morbidity-survey/adult-psychiatric-morbidity-survey-survey-of-mental-health-and-wellbeing-england-2014, accessed 19 November 2019.

Orrú M, Guitart X, Karcz-Kubicha M et al. 2013. Psychostimulant pharmacological profile of paraxanthine, the main metabolite of caffeine in humans. *Neuropharmacology*, 67, pp. 476–484.

Pritchard M. 2008. Disordered eating in undergraduates: Does gender role orientation influence men and women the same way? *Sex Roles*, 59, pp. 282–289.

Puhl R, Wharton C, Heuer C. 2009. Weight bias among dietetics students; implications for treatment practices. *Journal of the American Dietetic Association*, 109(3), pp. 438–444.

Quello SB, Brady KT, Sonne SC. 2005. Mood disorders and substance use disorder: A complex comorbidity. *Science Practice Perspectives*, 3(1), pp. 13–21.

RCP, RCPsych. 2013. *Smoking and Mental Health*. A joint report by the Royal College of Physicians and the Royal College of Psychiatrists Publisher. Suffolk: The Lavenham Press Limited.

Siennick SE, Widdowson AO, Woessner MK, Feinberg ME, Spoth RL. 2017. Risk factors for substance misuse and adolescents' symptoms of depression. *Journal of Adolescent Health*, 60(1), pp. 50–56.

Storther EL, Lemberg R, Stanford CE, Tuberviell D. 2012. Eating disorders in men: Underdiagnosed, undertreated, and misunderstood. *Eating Disorders*, 20(5), pp. 346–355.

Striley CLW, Griffiths RR, Cottler LB. 2011. Evaluating dependence criteria for caffeine. *Journal of Caffeine Research*, 1, pp. 219–225.

Sullivan MD. 2018. Depression effects on long-term prescription opioid use, abuse, and addiction. *Clinical Journal of Pain*, 34(9), pp. 878–884.

Virgo H. 2019. Eating Disorders are not just about weight #dumpthescales. https://www.refinery29.com/en-gb/2019/05/233545/dump-the-scales-eating-disorders-anorexia-petition, accessed 19 November 2019.

Wang JC, Hinrichs AL, Stock H et al. 2004. Evidence of common and specific genetic effects: Association of the muscarinic acetylcholine receptor M2 (CHRM2) gene with alcohol dependence and major depressive syndrome. *Human Molecular Genetics*, 13, pp. 1903–1911.

Watkins KE, Paddock SM, Zhang L, Wells KB. 2006. Improving care for depression in patients with comorbid substance misuse. *The American Journal of Psychiatry*, 163(1), pp. 125–132.

Weiss RD, Griffin ML, Greenfield SF, Najavits LM, Wyner D, Soto JA, Hennen JA. 2000. Group therapy for patients with bipolar disorder and substance dependence: Results of a pilot study. *Journal of Clinical Psychiatry*, 61(5), pp. 361–367.

Weltzin T. 2005. Eating disorders in men: Update. *Journal of Men's Health & Gender*, 2, pp. 186–193.

WHO. 2018. *International Classification of Diseases* 11th Revision (ICD 11). https://www.who.int/news-room/detail/18-06-2018-who-releases-new-international-classification-of-diseases-(icd-11), accessed 19 November 2019.

Young-Wolff KC, Kendler KS, Sintov ND, Prescott CA. 2009. Mood-related drinking motives mediate the familial association between major depression and alcohol dependence. *Alcoholism Clinical and Experimental Research*, 33, pp. 1476–86.

Chapter 6

The involvement of the father

Infant attachment

Whilst it is the woman who becomes pregnant, it is the couple who are expecting a baby. Expectant fathers' contributions have in the past been marginalised and any effort to capitalise on their motivations has been minimal. The antenatal period is a prime time to educate fathers on their important contribution and to encourage them to engage with the pregnancy. Involving them in the antenatal procedures, acquiring their attitudes to childbirth and child rearing as well as helping them to support their partners' breastfeeding, can all have positive outcomes.

Although the various means of maternal-infant attachment have been studied at length, there has been little research on the father-infant attachment and how his atypical behaviour can affect the development of the infant. Some studies, however, apply a methodology that is best suited to maternal-infant outcomes (Milford et al. 2006, Schoppe-Sullivan et al. 2006, Madigan et al. 2011, Brown et al. 2018).

It may be difficult for the father not to interpret the feelings of elation, preoccupation and self-absorption that the mother may be experiencing following childbirth, as her being distant, selfish and vague towards the father if he is unable to fully comprehend her situation. He may feel isolated, irrelevant and alone. While the mother is experiencing joy, the father may be more pragmatic, considering the strain of extra financial pressures, the sleepless nights and the unprecedented levels of responsibility that will ensue. However, without intervention, these negative thoughts can permeate throughout the pregnancy and the joy of being a father lost. Therefore, communication is the key. Having realistic expectations about his role and expectations can help assuage feelings of uselessness or hopelessness. Talking through the real fears that are felt would be beneficial. Naturally these will superimpose on the emotional fears about not being prepared and not being a 'good enough' father.

It may be easy for the mother to dismiss these comments, but, particularly if the father is already suffering from a depressive disorder or illness, then listening to his concerns and working together on a plan for the future, can help to alleviate any doubts he may have. It is worth reminding the father to list all the good and bad things about the pregnancy, followed by the positive and negative outcomes once the infant is born. This will help to put his thoughts into perspective.

Observing and participating in the whole process of the pregnancy can help the father to be a significant part of the progression. Health practitioners often comment on the lack of fathers attending antenatal classes even though they are available at convenient times for working men. Addressing why this occurs has flagged up the following reasons. Fathers are less likely to attend because they feel the classes are not aimed at them, but women. Some may feel intimidated, particularly if the women in attendance are in the majority. Timings are also an issue, as although there are flexible working hours, often it is difficult to have time off work. Another excuse is they have responsibility for the care of the other children in the home.

There is the assumption that women are experts on pregnancy and infants and the partner will be capable of managing any of the problems which may occur. However, when there is the realisation that both partners are equally ignorant of child-rearing practices, it is easier for both to share their own fears and expectations of the pregnancy, labour and developing infant (Smyth et al. 2015, Lerardi et al. 2018).

The father's perspective is different from the mother's. He does not go through the physiological changes, but he may encounter the same emotional responses. Learning about the intricacies of the labour and birthing process gives fathers a greater understanding and, in a men-only group, allows them to ask specific questions that may make them feel uncomfortable in a mixed gender group. Equally, if men were allowed to discuss any potential risks during the labour, to prepare them for a traumatic birth or complications with the infant, this would alleviate any reservations they may have about discussing perceived distressing events in front of their partner. The emphasis is about mutual support and recognising that both parents need encouragement and endorsement throughout the whole pregnancy.

Some fathers who attended classes have claimed their experience was not as positive or helpful in preparing them for their role as birth partners or indeed in parenthood. Others felt they would be unprepared if a complication at the birth arose. The common finding was that men would prefer a focus on their individual needs (Smyth et al. 2015). It is therefore preferable to have male-only antenatal classes where men can ask stupid questions or make comments without fear of reprisal from their partners.

Male only antenatal classes are already in existence, though currently they are greatly in the minority. These classes are focussed on and tailored to the needs of men. They concentrate on the physical elements of changing nappies, sleep techniques, the importance of play, soothing and bathing infants. There is also information on the brain development and the impact of stress and stimulation on the developing baby brain.

The level of the depression may be such that the sense of any low mood or disinterest may jeopardise the father's interactions with the pregnancy. He may withdraw or isolate himself from social settings and some of his perceived responsibilities. If his partner or the health professional is aware of his mental health history this will be the time to consider him being prescribed medication to help him cope with the ensuing pressures (Madigan et al. 2011).

During pregnancy it is important that the father's involvement continues from the very start. Fathers tend to develop close emotional ties with their infant around three days post-partum and invest and sustain their interest with the infant during this period (Bronte-Tinkew et al. 2007). This requires thought and support on the process of pregnancy, not only from a biological perspective, but from an emotional and behavioural standpoint. Support can be vital if the father is aware, not only of the consequences of a possible physical illness, but also of a mental disorder or illness. An awareness of his own mental health is key to understanding the contributions he can make and the limitations because he cannot.

Often the father may be lacking in confidence when trying to bond with his new-born infant and yet this is an integral part of parenting. There are numerous suggestions how to achieve this but for some men, the idea is overwhelming. It should be a natural progression in fatherhood and health professionals can be key in helping the father achieve a successful engagement with his child. When advising fathers on attachment issues, it is important to understand that the father is in control of his own emotions and the way in which he manages them. The father who did not experience a secure attachment bond as an infant may find it more challenging to connect with their infant. It becomes an additional task if the father is also depressed, but not insurmountable.

As the infant's nervous system is independent, it produces differing needs for the infant which sometimes makes it difficult to interpret the infant's emotions. Loving an infant is not the same as securing attachment. This requires insight and work. The whole successful experience releases endorphins which help to energise and motivate. For the depressed father, securing attachment is even more important as the rewards of a secure relationship with his infant will help him to have confidence in his ability to parent and to experience love. Often the attachment is with the primary parent, who may be the mother, but the father is able to benefit too.

There is copious literature on secure attachment and bonding but the meaning is sometimes obscure. It is defined as a unique emotional relationship between the infant and the carer (or father). The creation of this bond is designed by nonverbal communication. It is about responding to and understanding the meaning of the infant's cues. This can be translated as the types of movement the infant makes to indicate that they are fractious or happy. The gestures that demonstrate frustration or pleasure and understanding and differentiating between the infant's sounds of joy, pain and hunger (Madigan et al. 2011, Appleton et al. 2016, Brown et al. 2018).

There are specific cues which indicate that the infant is cold or needs to be comforted. These may include adjusting the position of their body or moving limbs in response to a voice. The facial expression may also change. When the appropriate response is made, by either sensitive, tender touching, rocking or is pacified with soothing music, then the infant becomes relaxed and the expressions and movements diminish.

Practical activities to nurture secure attachment include maintaining eye contact and calmly talking or singing whilst bottle feeding or changing the nappy. Reading out loud in a comforting manner or playing games, like peekaboo, poking the tongue out or blowing bubbles can help the infant to mimic the father's movements and help to secure attachment. Frequent touching and comforting the infant helps them both to emotionally interconnect. Making and taking the time to be with the child is important. The demanding child can be placated if there is a commitment to a time and place where they can both share space together. This works well if the father has to work or has a particular task to do. It can be given a name, like 'dad and daughter' time. The child will then know there is a period when they can be exclusively together.

Over time this security helps the infant to gain the necessary skills to develop and sustain relationships throughout their life. The brain is stimulated to not only develop socially, but is able to expand emotionally, intellectually and physically. It provides a platform for future self-awareness, empathy and healthy emotional wellbeing and relationships.

There may be doubt about the ability to read the infant's cues, and parents worry that they have misinterpreted them. There are several reasons why this may happen. Infants who appear hyper alert or move about wildly can be overtired, yet the misunderstanding is that they may want to play, when often they are signalling that they just need to sleep. Perhaps the infant is poorly or teething and is too preoccupied to engage with anything. This is termed a 'disconnection' and can be repaired the next time there is an appropriate response to a cue. If, however, the infant's needs are not met, then the infant develops feelings of insecurity and has mixed messages about other people's responses. This leads to confusion and difficulty in relating to others as the infant grows.

Exploring positive self-regard with empathetic responses, which is a psychological prerequisite for a healthy mind, can help the father to achieve his full potential. Encouraging and supporting him to engage with the infant he loves will help to expel the doubts he may have about his fathering skills.

What is known is that fathers tend to engage in more play than caring for the infant during infancy and early childhood. His sensitivity during his interactions with the infant can be a strong predictor of the infant's attachment during later childhood and adolescence. Stay-at-home fathers are now on the increase and the amount of time fathers now spend caring for the children has raised significantly (Milford et al. 2006, Appleton et al. 2016).

With verbal communication it is important to set realistic goals. These should include the father being a better listener, taking the time to be aware of what is being said without interrupting, and avoiding advice. The child should be valued and this can be highlighted by praise and encouraging words. Understanding the consequences of ill temper can be cathartic. It will be harmful to humiliate or mock the child; therefore, the father should be advised to wait until he is calm before addressing issues that may be of concern, as negative comments are damaging. Trust is a solid marker, as it allows the child to talk to and confide in the father without consequences.

Teenage girls are more likely to experience depression, which is even more intense in boys, if their father left at an early age. Those girls whose fathers left before they were five years of age were more likely to be depressed than those whose father left from the ages of five to ten years. This suggests that older children have time to develop more coping mechanisms and support networks outside the family to include friends (Culpin et al. 2013). Unconditional love is a powerful yardstick and to love a child because of who they are, not what they should be is a powerful emotion.

Other means of engaging the father include helping with breastfeeding, pram walking and baby massage. Although breastfeeding is the reserve of the mother, there may be times when bottle feeding is necessary. Encouraging the father to hold the infant in the same position as the mother would whilst breastfeeding; close to his chest, enables both he and the infant to gaze into each other's eyes. The infant is able to recognise his father's features and this helps to create the bond between the two. Encouraging regular involvement in the infant's routine of feeding, sleeping and nappy changing ensures the father is as much a part of the family as the mother.

Many fathers are now seen carrying infants in a sling or papoose. Equally we observe single fathers pushing prams and pushchairs around parks and shopping centres. The design of pushchairs which have the infant facing forwards away from the 'pusher' appears to be diminishing, as they are increasingly designed with the infant facing the 'pusher'; this allows greater interaction between the two.

One of the recommended therapies for attaining closer attachment with the infant and also for the father is baby massage. This has been popular for many years and was based on the theory that when human skin touches human skin it reduces the production of cortisol. This helps to decrease parental anxiety and can enhance the relationship between father and infant (Cheung et al. 2011). The more the father interacts with the infant, the more the levels of nurturing and sensory stimulation increase (Chen et al. 2017).

Baby massage

Skin-to-skin contact is the main component of baby massage as the emotions are communicated through touch. It is important that the activity takes place in a safe and secure environment. The infant is dried, laid onto a towel or blanket, and it is important that the activity takes place in a safe and secure environment. It can happen whenever an infant needs comfort or calming. With the infant lying on their front, using the fingertips, thumbs or palms, the baby can be massaged symmetrically down both sides of the body. Circular motions are used on the head, face and neck, with longer strokes along the infant's back, legs and feet. The infant is then placed on their back and the process repeated. Whilst this activity is being performed, the father is encouraged to talk to the infant, paying attention to the motions which give the infant the most pleasure and adapting their style accordingly.

Cullen et al. (2006) clarified these findings and requested fathers to massage their infants for fifteen minutes each evening for a month. A slightly different technique was used, by lightly stroking the infant's face and then using baby massage oil to 'milk' the legs. The emphasis was on massaging the whole body with criss-cross and circular motions. The techniques are simple, but need to be taught by an experienced practitioner in order to reap the full benefit, not only for the infant, but for the father to gain confidence and recognise if what he is performing is therapeutic and enjoyable. The main benefits are that it calms and relaxes both parent and infant by regulating the infant's heart rate, breathing and temperature. It stimulates the infant's digestive system, and protects against infection by enabling the colonisation of the parent's friendly bacteria onto the infant's skin (Fenwick 2001, Unicef 2019).

It is thought that the skin-to-skin attachment initiates strong, instinctive behaviours. The need to touch is innate in all humans, and the parent has the powerful urge to soothe the new-born infant. In fathers, this appears to create lower anxiety and depressive symptoms, which is important for better attainment of the parenting role (Huang et al. 2019). The loss of parental proximity and the ability to soothe and stimulate the infant are some of the potent stressors in early life. Studies have found that this type of neglect shows atypical patterns of diurnal hypothalamus, pituitary and adrenal activity (HPA Axis). There are lower levels of cortisol during the morning. In order to modulate this, the infant need to feel safe and that can be achieved by the closeness of the skin-to-skin contact (Scholz & Samuels 1992, Coyne 2017, Angelhoff et al. 2018).

However, there has been reluctance on the part of fathers to participate in any classes, despite the recommendations for health care practitioners. There are also some concerns around the actual massage activity, in both mothers and fathers, but with sensitive explanations highlighting the therapeutic values for both fathers and their infants; it has proved to be a beneficial and constructive pursuit (Mackereth & Tipping 2003).

Breastfeeding and the role of fathers

Breastfeeding mothers who have strong social support from their partner are more likely to initiate and continue breastfeeding (Brown & Davies 2014). In previous generations fathers took a step back when infant feeding was involved, rarely becoming concerned with breastfeeding methods and seldom prepared to make up bottles of formula milk. With the differing role of the father there is probably more reason for the father to be involved in the process and therefore a need for him to also be fully informed and supported. In recent studies, fathers have indicated that they would like to become more involved and more supportive (Sherriff et al. 2009, Sherriff and Hall 2011). Parents, particularly mothers, who have sufficient information about the processes of breastfeeding feel more informed and confident

(Brown et al. 2011), whilst mothers who have the support of their partner feel more capable and competent when making their breastfeeding decisions (Mannion et al. 2013). However, there has been criticism levied at health professionals for excluding fathers from anything 'baby-led'. This includes antenatal classes where information on breastfeeding is often an integral part of the courses (McQueen et al. 2011). There is overwhelming research to indicate that breastfeeding is best for the infant, making the supportive role of the father even more important. Breastfeeding brings its own challenges for the mother, making it more difficult for the father to become wholly involved, and he can often feel excluded from the whole experience (de Montigny & Lacharite 2004).

Story of a father's experience of breastfeeding

When Mike heard he was going to be a father for the first time, he was ecstatic. He had been brought up in care and this was his first real relationship. He was going to have his own family and he was going to give his baby the best start in life. He and his partner rented a flat in the town and nearer the delivery date, started to equip the nursery.

His partner had decided to breastfeed the infant but Mike was not very keen on this decision because he felt he couldn't be involved, but joked that at least he would be able to have a good night's sleep. However, he recognised it was her choice, as she had read so much about it and attended all the antenatal classes. He also felt it would be good for the baby as he was familiar with phrase 'breast is best' and knew it would be the right thing to do. As the family finances were tight, he recognised that breastfeeding was a cheaper option as bought milk was so expensive.

His partner found difficulty with breastfeeding. The baby didn't seem to suck properly and struggled at the breast. His partner cried and it was not long before Mike found himself suggesting his son was fed with formula milk. The midwife came and spoke with his partner but Mike felt it wasn't his place to be in the room with them as he felt it was women's business. Mike felt he was being isolated from both his partner and child and that the focus was on them alone. His son was receiving more of his partner's attention than he was and what was difficult was that his son and his partner seemed very comfortable together.

His desperation to help only made his partner irritable. The more he suggested an alternative as in formula feeding, the crosser she got. It appeared he had little choice and his suggestions did not matter. He tried to ask his partner to explain stuff, but he was ashamed because he felt that he should know.

Mike asked how he could help and was told to support his partner by doing some housework. Mike tried to help around the home. He washed and tidied up the clothes and hoovered, but his partner did not seem to appreciate it, as all she seemed to do was breastfeed. His son was feeding every hour and not only did it compromise any time with his partner but it exhausted Mike too

Mike desperately needed someone to talk to but his foster parents lived miles away, and he was separated from any close family. He felt embarrassed talking with his friends and when he looked online there were few specific videos, and most portrayed other women's breasts, which made Mike feel very uncomfortable. Mike was illiterate limiting his access to appropriate literature. When he did manage to get some leaflets, he found they were all directed at women and mostly written in a language he did not understand.

Mike started to resent the baby and quarrels with his partner became more intense. Mike became anxious as he realised his dream of a happy family was diminishing. He felt sad, alone and a rubbish father. He started drinking and left his partner with all the child care.

Whilst in the club and slightly inebriated, Mike chatted with a health worker who listened to his feelings of inadequacy and helplessness. He would never have spoken about his partner's breasts if he was sober. The worker suggested he spoke with the health visitor.

Mike plucked up the courage and contacted the health visitor and for once in a long time did not feel patronised. He was given tips on how to be more effective in his parenting by recognising the importance of his role and the significance of being supportive.

It has been recorded that fathers require more robust information on breastfeeding (Brown & Davies 2014). They need positive evidence about the extensive research into the benefits of breastfeeding, not just that it was 'best'. Specific details and demonstrations on breastfeeding solutions would help the father to understand the anatomy and physiology of mother and infant. Fathers should be forewarned about the potential challenges they may both encounter. The amount of time required for feeding may be minimised if fathers are unaware of the periods consumed in both the preparation and feeding times. Equally it may help if they know this occurs for only a short period of time.

The father's competencies, should be recognised and not patronised as something that they do not require, as it is the mother's territory. The father should be allowed be a part of the informed decision process. A joint decision can minimise the mother feeling guilty because of her choice of feeding. The father should discuss with, rather than tell his partner what he thinks is the best method, as there is the danger that increased involvement from the father can lead to feeding cues being missed, separation of the mother and infant or increased bottle use. This can lead to a reduced milk supply and in some cases ceasing breastfeeding altogether (Thulier & Mercer 2009). However, it is also possible that a mother chooses to formula feed to please both herself and her partner, allowing the father to become more involved in the infant's care (Brown et al. 2011).

Strategies should be in place to alleviate any difficulties in breastfeeding and extra support alerted if the mother requires respite. Embarrassment and shame also need to be addressed. The breast is often viewed as a sexual object, and mothers may feel uncomfortable discussing this within a group of mixed genders.

This may prohibit the presence of the father, but it remains a subject that should be taken into account. There may be cultural contexts that disallow the father from looking at, or being involved in any breastfeeding activity. Fathers may benefit from having the opportunity to read about or talk to fathers who have overcome their embarrassment.

Mood changes in the mother should be recognised, not challenged nor taken personally, but listened to and addressed. Equally the father should be aware of his mood and how his anxiety and or depression can have a negative impact on the mother. Health professionals are currently more aware of the challenges faced by parents, and time should be made to fully discuss queries and anxieties to ensure successful outcomes for the mother, father and infant.

References

Angelhoff C, Blomqvist YT, Helmer CS, Olsson E, Shorey S, Frostell A. 2018. Effect of skin-to-skin contact on parents' sleep quality, mood, parent-infant interaction and cortisol concentrations in neonatal care units: Study protocol of a randomised controlled trial. *Paediatrics BMJ Open*, 6(7), p. e021606.

Appleton R, Douglas H, Rheeston M. 2016. Taking part in 'Understanding Your Child's Behaviour' and positive changes for parents, *Community Practitioner*, 89(2), pp. 42–48.

Bronte-Tinkew J, Ryan S, Carrano J, Moore KA. 2007. Resident fathers' pregnancy intentions, prenatal behaviors, and links to involvement with infants. *Journal of Marriage and Family*, 69(4), pp. 977–990.

Brown A, Davies R. 2014. Fathers' experiences of supporting breastfeeding: Challenges for breastfeeding promotion and education. *Maternal and Child Nutrition*, 10(4), pp. 510–526.

Brown A, Raynor P, Lee M. 2011. Maternal control of child-feeding during breast and formula feeding in the first 6 months post-partum. *Journal of Human Nutrition and Dietetics*, 24(2), pp. 177–186.

Brown GL, Mangelsdorf SC, Shigeto A, Wong MS. 2018. Associations between father involvement and father–child attachment security: Variations based on timing and type of involvement. *Journal of Family Psychology*, 32(8), pp. 1015–1024.

Chen E-M, Gau M-L, Liu C-Y, Lee T-Z. 2017. Effects of father-neonate skin-to-skin contact on attachment: A randomized controlled trial. *Nursing Research and Practice*, 2017, p. 8.

Cheung CD, Volk AA, Marini ZA. 2011. Supporting fathering through infant massage. *Journal of Perinatal Education*, 20(4), pp. 200–209.

Coyne Medical. 2017. The power of father infant massage. Nov. online. https://www.coyne medical.com › the-power-of-father-infant-massage, accessed 19 November 2019.

Cullen C, Field T, Escalona A, Hartshorn K. 2006. Father-infant interactions are enhanced by massage therapy, *Early Child Development and Care*, 164(1), pp. 41–47.

Culpin I, Heron J, Araya R, Melotti R, Joinson C. 2013. Father absence and depressive symptoms in adolescence. Findings for a UK cohort. *Psychological Medicine*, 43(12), pp. 2615–2626.

de Montigny F, Lacharite C. 2004. Fathers' perceptions of the immediate postpartum period. *Journal of Obstetric, Gynecologic, and Neonatal Nursing*, 33(3), pp. 328–339.

Fenwick P. 2001. Psychoneuroimmunology: The mind-brain connection. In: Peters D (Ed.), *Understanding the Placebo Effect in Complementary Medicine*. London: Churchill Livingstone, pp. 215–226.

Huang X, Chen L, Zhang L. 2019. Effects of paternal skin to skin contact in newborns and fathers after caesarean delivery. *Journal of Perinatal and Neonatal Nursing*, 33(1), pp. 68–73.

Lerardi E, Ferro V, Trovato A, Tambelli R, Crugnloa CR. 2018. Maternal and paternal depression and anxiety: Their relationship with mother-infant interactions at 3 months. *Archives of Women's Mental Health*, 19, pp. 1–7.

Mackereth PA, Tipping L. 2003. A minority report: Teaching fathers baby massage. *Complementary Therapies in Nursing and Midwifery*, 9(3), pp. 147–154.

Madigan S, Benoit D, Boucher C. 2011. Exploration of the links among fathers' unresolved states of mind with respect to attachment, atypical paternal behaviour, and disorganized infant-father attachment. *Infant Mental Health Journal*, 32(3), pp. 286–304.

Mannion C, Hobbs A, McDonald S, Tough S. 2013. Maternal perceptions of partner support during breastfeeding. *International Breastfeeding Journal*, 8(1), p. 4.

McQueen KA, Dennis C-L, Stremler R, Norman CD. 2011. A pilot randomized controlled trial of a breastfeeding self-efficacy intervention with primiparous mothers. *Journal of Obstetric, Gynecologic, and Neonatal Nursing*, 40, pp. 35–46.

Milford R, Kleve L, Lea J, Greenwood R. 2006. A pilot evaluation study of the Solihull approach. *Community Practitioner*, 79(11), pp. 358–362.

Scholz K, Samuels CA. 1992. Neonatal bathing and massage intervention with fathers, behavioural effects 12 weeks after birth of the first baby: The Sunraysia Australia intervention project. *International Journal of Behavioural Development*, 15(1), pp. 67–81.

Schoppe-Sullivan S, Diener M, Mangelsdorf S, Brown G, McHale J, Frosch C. 2006. Attachment and sensitivity in family context: The roles of parent and infant gender. *Infant and Child Development*, 15, pp. 367–385.

Sherriff N, Hall V. 2011. Engaging and supporting fathers to promote breastfeeding: A new role for health visitors? *Scandinavian Journal of Caring Sciences*, 25, pp. 467–475.

Sherriff N, Hall V, Pickin M. 2009. Fathers' perspectives on breastfeeding: Ideas for intervention. *British Journal of Midwifery*, 17(4), pp. 223–227.

Smyth S, Dale S, Murray K. 2015. Does antenatal education prepare fathers for their role as birth partners and for parenthood? *British Journal of Midwifery*, 23(5), pp. 336–342.

Thulier D, Mercer J. 2009. Variables associated with breastfeeding duration. *Journal of Obstetric, Gynecologic, and Neonatal Nursing*, 38, pp. 259–268.

Unicef UK. 2019. The baby friendly initiative. https://www.unicef.org.uk/babyfriendly/

Chapter 7

Treatment and management techniques

Management

Assessment and screening

Currently there is no universal assessment for fathers' mental health or emotional wellbeing and despite the recognition of the mental health problems in the perinatal period, there is no recommended screening tool. There is no appreciation of a common, shared language which fathers can use to express how they really feel. There may be the climate of embarrassment and ridicule and some may fear their emotions may be misinterpreted and assumptions made about their ability to parent (Wilkins & Kemple 2011).

Having an understanding that anxiety alters the outcomes for the child and knowing the deleterious impact of anxiety on not only the mother but the family, it is important that parents should be screened during the perinatal period. There is a consistent agreement among researchers that there is a need for an anxiety measure, which should be offered consistently and multiple times (Staneva et al. 2015).

There is sufficient evidence to suggest that the Edinburgh Postnatal Depression Scale (EPDS) can be used to assess both fathers and mothers (Cox et al. 1987, Bergström 2013, Edward et al. 2015, Gutierrez-Galve et al. 2015). The EPDS is used worldwide and has been translated into twenty-seven languages, which make it the most popular screening tool for postnatal depression in mothers; therefore, the transition to enable it to be used with all fathers should not prove difficult.

The EPDS is a one-dimensional tool designed to identify low mood and depression (Schetter & Tanner, 2012). From close examination of the actual questions from the practitioner, indicators for anxiety traits can be seen, particularly the questions enquiring about unnecessary blame and guilt. Statistically significant positive correlations between the EPDS and other self-report anxiety scales were recorded by several studies (Austin & Priest, 2010, Austin et al. 2014, Lefkovics et al., 2017). The 'Male Depression Risk Scale' (MDRS) had been designed as an assessment tool that is sensitive to the depressive symptoms of anger, risk-taking behaviours and substance misuse. However, it is not in common usage (Rice et al. 2013).

The Gotland Scale was developed by Martin et al. (2013) which explores more male-centred questions around the rates of lethargy, anger attacks and aggression, substance abuse and risk-taking behaviour. This assessment tool appeared to generate a more accurate measure of depression and demonstrated that the rates of depression, unlike previous work, were equivalent to the rates of women.

It makes sense that the ability and opportunity to assess mothers and fathers can only increase the identification and recognition of a mood disorder, particularly when this is followed up with the clinical interview. If the practitioner relies on clinical judgement alone, there is a chance they may never be quite certain that they have captured the real thoughts and feelings of the parent. This is supported by evidence which found an increase in the number of cases referred to specialist services (Darwin et al. 2015, Whitelock 2016).

Evidence has suggested that fathers prefer to discuss their physical rather than mental ill health. One study found that men felt more comfortable discussing their behaviours and physical signs of distress, including difficulty in concentrating at work or suffering from headaches (Darwin et al. 2017). Although the work has not been validated, anecdotal experiential evidence indicates that further investigation into the behaviour of fathers has proved to be effective in determining the ability of the father to talk more freely about how he feels and can resonate with his own interpretation of depression (Williams & Hanley 2019).

The following questions, together with the subsidiary queries, have elicited results, which have allowed the father to understand his thoughts and feelings.

1. Do you tend to avoid socialising with family and friends since your baby's birth? Subsidiary questions could include overworking? or isolation?
2. How did you feel about the birth experience? Subsidiary questions – did you feel panicky or out of control?
3. Would you say your intake of alcohol has increased since your baby's birth?
4. Has your cigarette smoking increased and can you tell why?

There is merit in a combination of the approaches, particularly if the parent presents with false negatives. In other words, the self-report scale is open to abuse, and parents wishing to hide or deny their thoughts and feelings can do so by wrongly answering the questions.

Good judgement allows the practitioner to challenge the answer, if it is contrary to what they would have anticipated, to ascertain, with a fuller explanation, why the father answered as he did.

Barriers

Much has been written on the reticence of men and fathers in particular, to engage with the health services (Thompson et al. 2004, Oliver et al. 2005, Stein 2018, Baldwin et al. 2018). Men are more likely to seek help with their physical rather than mental symptoms. Although stigma around mental health is diminishing the culture of hoping it will come to an end if left alone, self-medicating or perhaps it is better to leave it until it becomes intolerable, persists.

In the UK a mother is routinely visited by a health practitioner during the perinatal period, and often there is minimal contact with the father. There might be a multitude of reasons, but it is often assumed that the father does not want to engage as he feels or is made to feel that the visit is the remit of his partner and his baby. There are other reasons which may include why the father, despite paternity leave, prefers to remain out of the room. It might be that he is disinterested in his infant, he is working or the couple are separated and he lives somewhere else (Baldwin et al. 2018).

One study by Price (2018) found a proportion of fathers who engaged with health practitioners declined to be a part of the screening process, whilst others declined to complete the EPDS, despite there being evidence of anxiety and or depression. The low scores on the EPDS often did not reflect the mental health of the father, which questions whether they were significant false positives. One recent study found that screening for paternal depression is associated with lower costs and higher health effects. The screening intervention for fathers could be cost effective compared with not screening at all and would improve the quality of life for fathers (Asper et al. 2018).

Screening and assessment for alcohol abuse

It is postulated that there is a need to screen for alcohol abuse in fathers (Scott 2017). Work by Aertgeerts et al. (2001) explored the work of Seppa et al. (1998) who devised the five-shot questionnaire designed to ascertain drinking habits.

The five questions asked: How often do you have a drink containing alcohol? How many drinks containing alcohol do you have on a typical day when you are drinking? Have people annoyed you by criticising your drinking? Have you ever felt bad or guilty about your drinking? Have you ever had a drink first thing in the morning to steady your nerves or get rid of a hang-over? These may be simplified or the number decreased; another example of questions might be: Have you found you are drinking more than usual? What makes you want to drink? Do you feel better after drinking? Does drinking increase your confidence? How often do you get a hangover? How does this affect your relationship with your partner? What do you feel about yourself?

Assisting the father to explore his drinking habits can help him to understand his avoidance behaviours which prevent him from confronting his true feelings. Listening to the answers should determine ways in which the father uses alcohol to self-medicate. This may also be used to establish his usage of illicit drugs. The father may minimise or even deny his consumption, but asking the questions will help him focus on the amount he is drinking and how it impacts his life. Whatever the screening or assessment methods, it would be morally wrong to offer any such tool if no resources are available to treat, manage or support the father.

Types of treatments

As the awareness of mental health and illness grows, so does the 'popularity' and plethora of remedies, interventions, treatments, management strategies and psychopharmacological solutions.

The problem is there is no one-size-fits-all solution, and often it is a case of a tried and tested outcome for the individual. As discussed, there are various mechanisms for the assessment for paternal mental illness and disorders. It makes sense to check whether a father has symptoms of anxiety or depression before making a decision on the best course of action. So often, however, the health practitioner makes the decision for the father, or the father may have the preconception that the health practitioner will make the decision for him.

Talking therapies

Talking therapies are thought to be one of the most effective interventions designed to help the father express, explain and understand why he is feeling as he does and what he can do about it. The common belief is that self-care is selfish; however, when there is a feeling of wellbeing, there is more likelihood of being kind to oneself, which in turn translates to being kind to each other. Behavioural and cognitive interventions also have a sound background in the efficacy of treating anxiety disorders. A significant number of fathers improve following the therapies and maintain good health following the course of treatment.

The transition to fatherhood can be complex, demanding and take its toll on the hardiest of men, but at no stage should it be assumed by the health practitioner that he is able to fully cope. The father may be reluctant to engage with the health practitioner whom he may consider intrusive and whose input has been historically reserved for the mother. A comprehensive knowledge, however, and interest in paternal mental health, illness and disorders will help to break down barriers and challenges. As awareness increases and more personalities are breaking down the barriers by discussing their own mental health and the problems they have encountered, so is the stigma reducing. Whereas in past days it would have been an anathema to talk openly about problems, particularly those concerned with mental health, it is now becoming more acceptable.

In order to identify the father's mental health needs it is important to listen to him. To allow this to happen the basic requisites are for a trusting relationship to develop, and the time in which to listen to him. This need not take a long time to establish, as once he realises, he will not be judged or made fun of, the father will be confident that he can rely on the health practitioner for discretion and prudence.

The Mental Health Foundation (2016) states that 28% of men compared with 33% of women had not sought any medical help for a mental health problem. For a significant number of men, it sometimes takes over two years before they disclose how they are feeling. This suggests that in the meantime, to help them cope, they are more likely to consider other methods of self-medication/treatment rather than consult a health practitioner.

Part of the issue may be the language that is used when assessing mental health, which tends to be more suited towards women (Robertson & Baker 2017, Stein 2018). Use of more masculine expressions suitable for the traditional male roles will help to engage men more fully and help them feel as if their thoughts and feelings are uniquely masculine. The avoidance of the recognised medical terminology in this approach helps to break down communication barriers. The semantics of the phrase 'mental health' often cause confusion, and mental health should be viewed as good in the same vein as physical health. The word is 'healthy', *I feel healthy'* should apply to both mental and physical health.

However, 'mental health' which is often inferred as 'mental' or 'mad', is sometimes used as derogatory term, and perhaps there is mileage in considering alternative language. Terminology is important and useful when attempting to engage fathers. It is not about patronising or academic language but about the communication norms for the time and being clear on the type of vernacular which allows fathers to feel relaxed and listened to.

The words 'stress' or 'stressed out' are powerful and recognisable and can be interpreted in many ways to help the father identify what causes him to be stressed and what he can do alleviate stress. This can include the excess in substance habits, difficulties with sleep and aggressive behaviour (Stein 2018). Determining whether it is acute or long-term stress, can help the health practitioner to understand the impact it may have on the father.

The term emotional regulation or talking about anxiety and emotions are acceptable to the younger father but not necessarily the older, who may prefer the terms 'overwhelmed' or 'overloaded'.

Numerous studies have established that men sometimes prefer not be forced into a 'counselling position', and view it as less masculine and perhaps more as a more feminine trait, but would rather the session be, as they might see it, 'non-confrontational'. This might be achieved by initially talking with the man in a situation that suits him. Often men prefer to talk to each other when they are side by side as it precludes eye contact. It is not a priority to be able to read the other person, and he may not be interested in body posture, the way a woman might be, as women are more prone to orientate their bodies towards a conversation by leaning forward, touching, smiling and nodding their head to indicate they are listening. This scenario may be viewed as challenging, and the face-to-face talking, which women prefer, presents as competitive posturing and stances. This position enables the father to feel more comfortable and eliminates any sense of any competition (Connell 1995, Rush 2006, Brod 2013). This type of stance does have its disadvantages. It is difficult to analyse the other person's nonverbal communications as they would not be able to synthesise, interpret or understand facial gestures and body movements.

Often side-by-side conversations occur by accident or because of the environment, with strangers. As an example, there is a preference for men to stand together at the bar rather than sit at a table. Men are able to derive intimacy when they are watching rugby or football matches and converse side by side. It is worth being innovative in working out how to engage with the father in the first instance. Working at a task or walking together may help to prompt a conversation.

Active listening is not easy as health practitioners want to be prescriptive, by suggesting and advising the father. The answers are often obvious and the solutions straightforward, but for the father who may be in the depths of despair, they are not. It is he who has to makes sense of what is happening in his world and often just by being allowed to unravel his thoughts will help to understand the reasons for his distress. If helpful advice is given this can only reinforce his own inability to find an explanation for the way he is feeling. Listening and reflecting back what he has said can let the father know you have not only heard him but understand what he has said (Hanley 2015).

The health practitioner will already possess the necessary qualities of empathy and patience, which are vital skills in order to initiate any therapy. The process is one of listening, reflecting, paraphrasing and summarising.

A conversation can be started by, *'You seem to be fairly stressed and don't seem to be managing fatherhood as well as you usually do. Perhaps this is something we can talk about'? It's okay, take your time'.*

The father tells his story and the health practitioner listens. The next step is to reflect back or double check what he has said. This indicates that the practitioner has understood how he is feeling and what he thinks. This process is to prevent any misunderstandings and can confirm what has actually been said. For example, *'You say you think you are a bad father because you can't seem to console your son when he cries. You feel nervous when you are holding him and are afraid you will hurt him if you hold him too tight. You seemed angry when you were telling me this, am I right'?*

This enables the father to hear his own thoughts and feelings and to correct the interpretation if necessary, by suggesting he is not angry, but worried. He may suggest that he always feels worried but not just when he is holding his son. It is tempting to assure him he is a good father with, *'Don't be silly, everyone is worried when they try to calm a baby. I am sure you are a great father'.* Whereas this may sound helpful, it indicates that the father has not been really listened to, as he may feel like that because he has severe anxiety and unable to make his own decisions.

At the end of the session it is useful to summarise what the father has said. For example, *'You told me that you are worried about holding the baby because you are frightened you will hurt him. You also said you think you are a bad father as this is not the only thing you are not good at. You find yourself getting worked up at the slightest thing, sometimes getting angry. You have not spoken about this to anyone as you feel so ashamed but equally you are concerned that you will hurt your son. You are not sure if your wife has noticed but you will sit down with her tonight and ask her. You will also have a chat with your father as you think he may have felt the same about you. You recognise you are very anxious and will practice some deep breathing exercises and we will discuss how you got on next week'.*

It is probable that the father has not confronted his own anxieties or depression, therefore, allowing him to explore the reasons he feels and thinks as he does can be can be cathartic. This person-centered approach allows a rapport to develop and the contracted time between the father and the health practitioner ensures a mutual compliance. If this process takes place around the time of childbirth it has the ability to optimise the father's relationship with his partner, his infant and himself.

Keeping safe

As with all personal interactions, it is important not to become too familiar with the father; it should always be a therapeutic relationship. Keep safe. Private contact details should never be divulged, neither should personal details. Notes of the visits and interventions should always be kept. It is a therapeutic relationship and many issues will be shared; however, unless they are harmful or detrimental to their own wellbeing or that of their family, confidences should be respected. Something which was disturbing should always be shared with a supervisor or mentor.

Telephone communication

In the first instance, it might be easier for the father to have a telephone conversation. It has been argued that although health professionals recognise the father's mental health is important, it is also sometimes very difficult to engage with the father because of work commitments or perhaps the fact that he does not want to engage.

As one alternative it is worth suggesting a telephone call. This may be an old-fashioned technique in a world of social media, video conferencing and android apps, such as WhatsApp, but it allows a modicum of privacy and allows the health practitioner to listen rather than be distracted by the influence of visual images. However, this is not to say that talking with fathers is easy because it does not allow the ability to see their facial expressions, should something be discussed that may trigger a negative reaction.

Listening, as has been noted before, is a skill, and it is recommended that health practitioners receive training prior to undertaking any form of interviewing. It is also useful to initially and periodically, have a supervisor monitoring the calls. This will help to gain confidence and highlight any errors. There have been suggestions to consider, in the UK, teaming up with Australian helplines to support fathers who may be feeling vulnerable in the early hours of the morning. The timing corresponds with the afternoon in Australia, when support services are active. A reciprocal agreement could be made for Australian fathers who may need equal support in their early mornings.

Techniques

A dedicated phone number should be available to ensure safety and security. A personal number should never be used because of the risk of receiving a distressed text.

There should be minimal background noise to enable both to be heard clearly. A notepad should be available to write down any relevant information and to act as an aide memoire.

The father should always be asked a phone number on which he can be re-connected as a precaution against losing the mobile or land line signal.

It is important to talk with confidence and have an opening, rehearsed line, for example: *'Hello my name is John, what's yours? Thanks for taking the time to call me and how can I help you today'?*

Although it sounds obvious, there should be a beginning, middle and an end to the conversation, but often it is difficult to know where to start. It is important to be calm and patient. If the father hesitates, he should not be rushed but told to take his time. If he feels more comfortable, he can start in the middle! Initially it is beneficial to discuss whatever spontaneously comes into his mind. He should be allowed to talk freely but equally it is important to ensure the conversation does not go off track; to achieve this, reminding him of the initial problem should be sufficient. It is essential to ensure that everything that is said is heard correctly, therefore, seeking clarity and asking the father to repeat himself is acceptable. If an assumption is made and the father suspects he is not being listened to, this can jeopardise the rapport.

Having a solution to the problem is not always possible, but allowing the father to 'listen' to his own problems often allows him to make sense of what he said and as a result he is able to formulate his own solutions.

It is imperative that the father is not promised anything that is impossible to deliver. This is particularly important when discussing suicidal ideation or safeguarding, with any suggestion of keeping quiet or maintaining confidentiality. If the father is expressing suicidal thoughts, he must be directed to an appropriate helpline telephone number with instructions to contact it at the end of the phone call.

The last few minutes of the call are crucial, and to prevent fatigue of both parties, an agreed time limit should be established. When phone companies charge after one hour's usage, it is probably sensible to limit calls to an hour. The father should feel safe and be equipped with some solution to enable him to access the correct source of help.

Cognitive behavioural therapy (CBT)

One of the more effective therapeutic interventions is cognitive behavioural therapy (Cuijpers et al. 2013). This is used for an increasingly wide range of disorders.

There is evidence to suggest that there is a lack of support and treatments tailored specifically for men who have difficulty adjusting to fatherhood. With the limited available options, cognitive behavioural therapy appears to be more affective in supporting fathers with perinatal depression and anxiety. This is a psychosocial intervention which examines life situations, problems and difficulties, explores the reasons for any negative thinking and behaviours and attempts alter them to more positive responses. It is a combination of behavioural and cognitive psychotherapies. CBT focuses on the challenging and changing behaviours which limit the father's ability to function, because his thinking is mostly in negative terms. This thinking influences his belief system and ultimately the way he behaves.

The therapist is an integral part of the sessions and plays an active role by guiding the father. The emphasis is not on the cause of his problem but how he interprets it. The therapist tries to understand the father's lifestyle and teaches him how to compensate for any shortcomings in a constructive way. The importance of 'we are what we do' is stressed because the idea is to help the father to understand and to practice effective strategies to address the identified goals and help diminish his negative feelings. This helps him to learn ways in which he can process information and, in turn, can deliver coping mechanisms. Anecdotal evidence suggests that men find it easier to cope and focus on one particular factor at a time; this differs from women who are able to consider several factors and work with them simultaneously (Beck 2011, Otte 2011, O'Neal and Parry 2015). A course of CBT can take up to twenty sessions and may last from thirty–sixty minutes, depending on the therapist and the client.

Story of a father who had CBT

Graham was suffering from perinatal depression. He had not had a history of depression but the overwhelming stress he felt following the birth of his son seemed to 'tip him over the edge'. He had only sought help when his employer warned Graham he would be suspended if his work output did not improve. Graham had always prided himself on being one of the most sought after lawyers for his expertise. This threat caused him greater distress. He started having sleepless nights and stomach pains. When Graham reluctantly visited his doctor, he was prescribed antidepressants. Graham was appalled and suggested there was no way he would take any medication that would make him dopey, particularly as he had to have all his wits about him on his job.

The next course of action was a course of cognitive behavioural therapy. Graham was put on a waiting list, but this proved to be too long. Instead he decided to go privately and had his first session a few weeks later.

Initially, Graham was skeptical of the treatment, but felt he had no option but to attend.

Graham said: "I felt really uncomfortable during the original session. I just did not know what to expect, however as the course continued over the next eight sessions, I had a clear sense of what I was doing wrong and how I needed to alter my thinking processes.

For example, I really felt my boss had a downer on me. I began to notice that he was ignoring me when I passed him in the corridor. Normally he would acknowledge me but since I'd been feeling low, I thought it was his way of not confronting me, and he could avoid talking with me. I started to feel as if he was snubbing me, which made me feel even worse.

I found that I had no appetite, which was unusual because I was always ready for a sandwich. When I tried to eat, I just felt nauseated. I noticed I started to have stomach cramps and I generally felt bloated. Each time I saw my boss I found it easier to avoid him. I noticed I was planning my day so that I would have minimal contact with him.

So how did the CBT help? Well I was taught about how thoughts affect feelings which affect behaviour. I didn't know there was a difference, but it made sense. So, to reconstruct the example I just gave you. The therapist asked me to think about my reaction to my boss, but instead of thinking he was ignoring me, perhaps my boss was actually consumed with worry about something else.

There was I thinking about myself and me, and he was probably going through a tough time himself. Then I felt really sorry for him, perhaps he was feeling like me, but also afraid to show it? I felt a bit ashamed of my own thoughts, and this certainly made me want to make an effort to make sure he was okay. I made a point of asking him how he was. This took a lot of courage as I had spent so much time (in my mind anyway) avoiding him. To my surprise, my boss frowned and put his hand on my shoulder and sighed, 'not good'. He had been struggling with the company finances and was concerned that he would have to make someone redundant. He felt isolated and hoped he hadn't caused too much stress within the company.

With lots of practice, this experience has taught me to alter my thinking and to think positively before I allow any negative thoughts to permeate my brain. I can now eat normally and my sleep pattern is improving. I think that a combination of an improvement in both these has lifted my mood and I don't feel so overwhelmed."

The vicious cycle of self-blame, feelings of reproach and avoidance behaviour can be hard to break, but with support and understanding about why the father thinks, feels and behaves as he does, can help to change his world.

Cognitive behavioural therapy is not successful in all cases and may not suit everyone. For those fathers with special needs or complex mental health problems, it may be advisable to consider other forms of therapy. It focuses on the father's ability to change himself; it does not focus on the causes, which may include childhood experiences, and does not offer a fix-all situation, which may include the issues within the wider family. Although the therapist can offer support and advice there has to be a sense of commitment from the father. Family life may be constrained by the amount of time that has to be spent in therapy. Confronting emotions, coupled with anxieties, may prove too daunting for some.

It is, however, suitable and successful where medication alone has not worked. It can be completed in a relatively short time compared with other therapies. As it is highly structured it can be provided in different formats, which include group work, self-help books and apps. It continues to teach practical and useful strategies which can be used in everyday life, even when the treatment has been completed. There is still work to be done on the models of therapies which are based on father-specific and father-inclusive care, to ensure that fathers are able to be engaged with the services and gain benefits from them.

Resilience

Resilience is viewed as a defence mechanism, which enables fathers to thrive in the face of adversity. However, some of the approaches do not have a unilateral structure, making it difficult to determine how any one approach may be applied. The philosophy of resilience is enabling the father to have the capacity to quickly recover from any difficult situation he may encounter. It is grounded in his childhood and is influenced primarily by his childhood experiences and the impact they will have had on his personal life (Masten 2014). Personal resilience is thought to protect the father's psychological health and enables psychological positivity in the face of adversity and other significant challenges. It enables focus to be retained on what is important and to cope effectively with any challenge, providing it is not overwhelming for the father (Davydov et al. 2010).

Fostering the capacity in order to develop resilience involves looking after physical as well as mental health. Therefore, eating well, taking regular exercise and taking rest when appropriate, are all important factors. The regulation of cognitive emotions which are involved in preplanning, positive appraisal and the ability to ruminate less, contribute to the resilience of those with anxiety and depressive disorders.

Mindfulness

This therapy is increasing in popularity. It has roots in Buddhism and has been practiced for over 2,000 years. It was only in the late 1970s when a successful mindfulness-based stress reduction programme was devised and became responsible for reducing chronic pain, that it gained notoriety. During the early 2,000s, a mindfulness-based cognitive therapy for depression was developed to help prevent the relapse of depression (Segal et al. 2002).

Mindfulness seeks to achieve a relaxed, non-judgemental awareness of thoughts, feelings and sensations. It is an understanding of what is happening both inside and outside the body at each moment in time. It helps fathers learn to direct their attention to the experience as it unfolds rather than keeping it in their heads. Ruminating thoughts can easily consume the mind and can, if unchecked, take over, causing anxiety and depressed symptoms. Practice at this art eventually results in the ability to connect with the present moment by calmly being aware of thoughts, sensations and feelings and, in turn, being able to effectively manage them, and slowly they become less intrusive (Segal et al. 2002, Kabat-Zinn 2015). Clinical trials have found that mindfulness is as effective as antidepressants and can reduce the occurrence of depression by 40%–50% compared with other methods of treatment (NICE 2004).

Practice is the key, and making time to perform the technique each day for at least fifteen minutes or during periods of sleeplessness or stress, will help to focus the mind. It is recommended to sit calmly in a quiet place, breathe deeply, feeling the air course through the nose into the belly. Paying attention to the surroundings, quietly trains the mind to be aware, focus and filter. Whilst being in the moment, there is little opportunity to regret the past or worry about the future. Another time to practice this is when the father feels overwhelmed by his environment. This may involve him trying to do his tax returns, answer the phone and listen to the football results, whilst being in charge of a fretful infant. Breaking away from the situation and concentrating on a single object, for example a picture on the wall and consciously regulating breathing, helps to calm the mind. This may take less than ten minutes before he is able to return to the situation feeling in a more composed and tranquil state. When the father is more adept at mastering the technique, this is referred to as mindful mindfulness. Like physical exercise, mindfulness is a form of mental exercise, with similar gains. Once the benefits are realised it often inspires a lifelong function (Goleman & Davidson 2017).

Groups and support networks

Despite the complex needs of fathers during the postnatal period, groups are still designed exclusively for mothers. Unless he chooses to take parental leave, it is only during the two weeks paternity leave that the father has the opportunity to adjust to parenthood. This leaves a limited time for him to access services. However, if the father has been aware of the potential difficulties he may encounter, then this period is the ideal time for sourcing suitable groups or support networks.

Evidence suggests that therapeutic groups have a positive effect, largely because of the human intervention by voluntary or statutory agencies (MMHA 2019). The relationship formed in groups can lead to social interactions that help to satisfy the basic need to affiliate with others in a similar situation (Shaw 1976, Pitts 1995). It can improve self-esteem and the general mood state. Often when the group is orientated around an activity, it has been reported anecdotally, that the discussion is rated higher than the actual purpose of the group.

As the incidence of the 'stay at home father' has increased, so is the potential for developing groups specifically designed for men. Several have been created over the past few years, but it has taken enterprising individuals to cultivate and expand them. Those that work have established an inclusive environment, providing a therapeutic atmosphere in which fathers can connect, bond and have the confidence and security to openly discuss and share how they feel. Weekly meetings, which include the infant, however, are not as common; those which do, not allow some respite time for the father. The growth of some groups has enabled them to consider spending quality time away, by going camping, fishing or playing sports, such as golf.

Suggesting teenage fathers attend groups might be an anathema to some, and they would prefer to pursue informal sources of help on the internet. There are groups on Facebook which offer the opportunity for self-disclosure, feedback between posters, together with offers and recommendations for help. One study found the posters utilised adolescent Facebook groups, primarily to connect with those who might share a similar experience and to share information about available services (Lerman et al. 2016). However, Facebook posts and social media are often unregulated, but some of the content has the potential to utilise the exchange of evidenced- based information between groups to promote more traffic on- and offline.

There is a linkage between both physical and mental wellbeing and physical activities. Challenging and allowing the ability to take on a challenge that might otherwise be feared or rejected, allows fathers to build their confidence and self-esteem, knowing they are supported by others. It can also reduce negative thoughts and curtail destructive behaviour (thebookofman 2019).

References

Aertgeerts B, Buntinx F, Ansoms S, Fevery J. 2001. Screening properties of questionnaires and laboratory tests for the detection of alcohol abuse or dependence in a general practice population. *British Journal of General Practice*, 51, pp. 206–217.

Asper MM, Hallen N, Lindberg L, Mansdotter A, Carlberg M, Wells MB. 2018. Screening fathers for postpartum depression can be cost-effective: An example from Sweden. *Journal of Affective Disorders*, 241(1), pp. 154–163.

Austin M, Hanley J, Wisner K. 2014. Marcé international society position statement onpsychosocial assessment and depression screening in perinatal women. *Best Practice Research Clinical Obstetric Gynaecology*, 28(1), pp. 179–187.

Austin MP, Priest S. 2010. Depressive and anxiety disorders in the postpartum period: How prevalent are they and can we improve their detection? *Archives of Women's Mental Health*, 13(5), pp. 395–401.

Baldwin S, Malone M, Sandall J, Bick D. 2018. Mental health and wellbeing during the transition to fatherhood: A systematic review of first time fathers' experiences. *JBI Database of Systematic Reviews and Implementation Reports*, 16(11), pp. 2118–2191.

Beck JS. 2011. *Cognitive Behavior Therapy: Basics and Beyond*, 2nd ed. New York, NY: The Guilford Press, pp. 19–20.

Bergström M. 2013. Depressive symptoms in new first-time fathers: Associations with age, sociodemographic characteristics and antenatal psychological well-being. *Birth*, 40(1), pp. 32–38.

Brod H. 2013. Men's studies: A retrospective view. *Journal of Men's Studies*, 21(1), pp. 49–61.

Connell RW. 1995. *Masculinities*. Berkeley, CA: University of California Press.

Cox J, Holden J, Sarkovsky R. 1987. Detection of postnatal depression. Development of the 10-item Edinburgh postnatal depression scale. *British Journal of Psychiatry*, 150, pp. 782–786.

Cuijpers P, Sijbrandij M, Koole SL et al. 2013. The efficacy of psychotherapy and pharmacotherapy in treating depressive and anxiety disorders: A meta-analysis of direct comparisons. *World Psychiatry*, 12, pp. 137–148.

Darwin Z, Galdas P, Hinchliff S, Littlewood E, McMillan D, McGowan L, Gilbody S. 2017. Fathers' views and experiences of their own mental health during pregnancy and the first postnatal year: A qualitative interview study of men participating in the UK Born and Bred in Yorkshire (BaBY) cohort. *BMC Pregnancy Childbirth*, 17, p. 45.

Darwin Z, McGowan L, Edozien LC. 2015. Antenatal mental health referrals: Review of local clinical practice and pregnant women's experiences in England. *Midwifery*, 31(3), pp. e17–e22.

Davydov DM, Stewart R, Ritchie K, Chaudieu I. 2010. Resilience and mental health. *Clinical Psychology Review*, 30(5), pp. 479–495.

Edward KL, Castle D, Mills C, Davis L, Casey J. 2015. An integrative review of paternal depression. *American Journal of Men's Health*, 9(1), pp. 26–34.

Goleman D, Davidson R. 2017. *Altered Traits: Science Reveals How Meditation Changes your Mind, Brain and Body*. New York: Penguin Random House.

Gutierrez-Galve L, Stein A, Hanington L, Heron J, Ramchandani P. 2015. Paternal depression in the postnatal period and child development: Mediators and moderators. *Pediatrics*, 135(2), pp. e339–e347.

Hanley J. 2015. *Listening visits in Perinatal Mental Health*. Oxford: Routledge.

Kabat-Zinn J. 2015. Mindfulness. *Mindfulness*, 6(6), pp. 1481–1483.

Lefkovics E, Rigó J, Szita B, Talabér J, Kecskeméti A, Kovács I, Baji I. 2017. Relevance of anxiety in the perinatal period: Prospective study in a Hungarian sample. *Journal of Psychosomatic Obstetrics and Gynecology*, 3, pp. 1–8.

Lerman BI, Lewis SP, Lumley ML, Gorgan GJ, Hudson CC, Johnson E. 2016. Teen depression groups on Facebook: A content analysis. *Journal of Adolescent Research*, 32(6), pp. 719–741.

Martin LA, Neighbors HW, Griffith DM. 2013. The experience of symptoms of depression in men vs women: Analysis of the National Comorbidity Survey Replication. *JAMA Psychiatry*, 70(10), pp. 1100–1106.

Masten A. 2014. Global perspectives on resilience in children and youth. *Child Development*, 85(1), p. 6.

Maternal Mental Health Alliance.org (MMHA). 2019. A charity campaigning for better services for women with perinatal mental health. https://maternatalmentalhealthalliance.org

Mental Health Foundation. 2016. Fundamental facts about mental health. Prevention is at the heart of what they do as the best way to deal with a crisis is to prevent it happening in the first place. http://www.mentalhealth.org.uk

National Institute for Clinical Excellence. 2004. *Depression: Management of Depression in Primary and Secondary Care*. Clinical Guideline 23. http://www.nice.org.uk/CG023NICEguideline

Oliver MI, Pearson N, Coe N, Gunnell D. 2005. Help-seeking behaviour in men and women with common mental health problems: Cross-sectional study. *British Journal of Psychiatry*, 186, pp. 297–301.

O'Neal EM, Parry MM. 2015. Help-seeking behavior among same-sex intimate partner violence victims: An intersectional argument. *Criminology, Criminal Justice Law and Society*, 16, pp. 51–67.

Otte, C. 2011. Cognitive behavioural therapy in anxiety disorders: Current state of the evidence. *Dialogues in Clinical Neuroscience*, 13(4), pp. 413–421.

Pitts F. 1995. Comrades in adversity: The group approach. *Health Visitor*, 68(4), pp. 144–145.

Price R. 2018. A project to support fathers with paternal depression. *Journal of Health Visiting*, 6(8), pp. 380–386.

Rice SM, Fallon BJ, Aucote HM, Möller-Leimkühler AM. 2013. Development and preliminary validation of the male depression risk scale: Furthering the assessment of depression in men. *Journal of Affective Disorders*, 151(3), pp. 950–958.

Robertson S, Baker P. 2017. Men and health promotion in the United Kingdom: 20 years further forward? *Health Education Journal*, 76(1), pp. 102–113.

Rush C. 2006. *Guy Talk vs Girl Talk; The Secret to Really Understanding each Other*. New York: Cosmopolitan, 240(6), pp. 140–143.

Schetter CD, Tanner L. 2012. Anxiety, depression and stress in pregnancy: Implications for mothers, children, research, and practice. *Current Opinion in Psychiatry*, 25(2), p. 141.

Scott R. 2017. Exploring health visitor's perspectives of screening parents for alcohol misuse. *Journal of Health Visiting*, 5(5), pp. 226–234.

Segal ZV, Teasdale JD, Williams JM, Gemar MC. 2002. The mindfulness-based cognitive therapy adherence scale: Inter-rater reliability, adherence to protocol and treatment distinctiveness. *Clinical Psychology and Psychotherapy*, 9(2), pp. 131–138.

Seppa K, Lepisto J, Sillanaukee P. 1998. Fiveshot questionnaire on heavy drinking. *Alcoholism Clinical and Experimental Research*, 22, pp. 1788–1791.

Shaw ME. 1976. *Group Dynamics: The Psychology of Small Group Behavior*, 2nd ed. New York: McGraw Hill.

Staneva A, Bogossian F, Pritchard M, Wittkowski A. 2015. The effects of maternal depression, anxiety, and perceived stress during pregnancy on preterm birth: A systematic review. *Women and Birth*, 28(3), pp. 179–193.

Stein C. 2018. *Mind Your Language: How Men Talk about Mental Health*. London: Men's health Forum.

The Book of Man. 2019. Men's media brand offering advice and inspiration to the modern man, from mental health, relationships and emotions to opinion and entertainment. https://www.thebookofman

Thompson A, Hunt C, Issakidis C. 2004. Why wait? Reasons for delay and prompts to seek help for mental health problems in an Australian clinical sample. *Social Psychiatry and Psychiatric Epidemiology*, 39(10), pp. 810–817.

Wilkins D, Kemple M. 2011. *Delivering Male effective Practice in Male Mental Health*. London: Men's Health Forum.

Williams M, Hanley J. 2019. The tool for measuring postnatal wellbeing in men. Conference presentation, 27th June. Oxford, England: Oxford Brookes University.

Whitelock A. 2016. Why do health visitors screen mothers and not fathers for depression in the postnatal period? *Journal of Health Visiting*, 4(6), pp. 312–321.

Chapter 8

Lifestyle factors

As well as the biological and psychosocial studies, research has concentrated on other factors involving everyday lifestyle factors which influence mood and the impact the neurotransmitter processes, anti-inflammatory and HPA axis and the immune-inflammatory pathways. The three contenders are diet, exercise and sleep, and it is now recognised that these have a somewhat profound effect on occurrence of depression.

There have been significant changes in the traditions in which food is consumed. Modern houses are often too small to accommodate the dining room with the required accoutrements for a dining experience, and meals on laps has become the norm. The supposition was that mothers were responsible for cooking the meals, but market research has indicated a gender reversal with almost half of fathers now preparing meals with over a quarter taking on sole responsibility. It has been suggested that fathers view their culinary skills as a sign of status. They are also keen to teach their children to cook. These actions have been challenged by some feminists who argue that men take the stance that cooking is a leisure activity and not proper 'work', a domain traditionally reserved for women (Szabo 2013).

The current trend in obesity has been blamed on a stressed lifestyle where time is of the essence and prepackaged convenience foods provide an alternative to the home-cooked meal. Technical innovations in vacuum packaging and improved preservatives have enabled manufacturers to mass prepare food cheaply and centrally for immediate consumption (Hanley 2017). This is compounded by the accessibility of fast food restaurants which, even in rural areas, are no further than a twenty-minute drive away and usually placed close to a motorway or road near the drive home. These outlets offer processed foods and meats which if taken in excess quantities have been associated with an increased risk of depression up to six years later (Sanchez-Villegas et al. 2012).

Diet

Studies have linked the high intake of sugary foods and beverages in the diet to an increase in obesity amongst the younger generations (Dimitrios et al. 2016). Some have connected this to an increase in the number of presentations of depressive disorders (Goldney et al. 2010). It has long been accepted that a 'Mediterranean diet' consisting of fish, vegetables and olive oil has been an indicator of a healthy lifestyle, but in recent years it has been noted that this intake has been a protector against depression. One study suggested that a greater adherence to a Mediterranean diet, moderate alcohol intake and daily tea drinking appear to have a beneficial effect on depressive symptoms in older adults (Masana et al. 2018). Studies have indicated that the less meat and the more vegetables and fresh fruits consumed, the lesser the risk of suffering from depression (Beezhold & Johnston 2012, Ford et al. 2013). Other studies have found that high fat and sugary junk food diets in adolescents have also been associated with depressive symptoms (Monster 2018). One study made connections between poverty, insufficient nutrients and the increase in depression (German et al. 2011).

The association between polyunsaturated fatty acids, particularly the omega-3 essential fatty acids, including eicosapentaenoic acid (EPA) and docosahexaenioc acid (DHA) and depressive symptoms has been of interest to scientists. High levels are found in fish oils, cold water fatty fish—for example, salmon, mackerel and herring—and nuts and seeds. Research trials found that when the EPA was supplemented in the diet, there appeared to be a beneficial effect to mental health (Sublette et al. 2011).

In light of the growing evidence to support the fact that some forms of depression are linked to a chronic low-grade inflammation of the body, the diet also plays a leading role. The levels of inflammatory markers of those suffering with depression are higher than those who are not depressed. This can be linked to those suffering from influenza, where the symptoms of poor sleep patterns, the inability to concentrate and feeling miserable are also linked to depressive symptoms. The study was only able to establish an association between depression and inflammation but not causation (Cepeda et al. 2016).

The immune system is activated when a foreign object enters the body. In the case of nutrients this can be an invading microbe, plant pollen or a chemical. This triggers an immune response which is termed inflammation; this is programmed to protect the body, as in any inflammatory response. There are anti-inflammatory foods, which it is claimed are able to reduce the risk of illness, whilst an over excess of the wrong foods, could accelerate the inflammatory disease process (Hu 2018). It has been suggested that limiting or avoiding certain foods can decrease the inflammation. These include refined carbohydrates which are found in white bread and pastries, fried foods, red and processed meats—for example burgers and sausages—margarine and sugary drinks. These foods are also linked with depressive symptoms. The foods which are anti-inflammatory include the Mediterranean foods of olive oil, tomatoes, fish, salads and nuts (Hu 2018).

The quality of the diet is important because of the effect it can have on the production of the monoamines such as serotonin and dopamine and the influences on the receptor sensitivity and neurotransmitter transporters within the brain. There have been diets of extremes in animal studies whereby they have been subjected to high carbohydrate or protein diets, which have affected the serotonin levels in the brain. When significant amounts of carbohydrates have been consumed over a short period of time, this has been found to increase the levels of tryptophan and serotonin in the brain. Other nutrients which were altered in those with major depression and influenced neurotransmitter production are folic acid, zinc, vitamin B12 and iron (Lopresti et al. 2015).

It appears that the extra fat cells release toxins that probably interfere with the neurotransmitters and hormonal system and this, in turn, has implications for mental health. Brain science should enable an understanding of the importance of diet, and yet the limitations of a healthy diet are inevitable, particularly for the father who finds himself in a hectic lifestyle, dictated by work and home commitments. Television adverts that portray the father as having both the time and energy to create a sumptuous meal are probably fantasy, and the reality is more reliance on fast foods. Naturally all of the advice for healthy eating is preventative, but what happens when the father's mood is so depressed that he is unable to consider eating at all?

The advertising industry has taken on the mantle, and there are more adverts featuring fathers and their role as an integral part of the family. However, with the inference on the young slim lady eating yoghurt, a father eating a healthy meal is yet to be highlighted.

One of the activators for dopamine, which affects the pleasure and reward centres in the brain, is the availability of food. It is suggested that overweight men have impairments in dopamine pathways, blunted through the constant exposure to sugary and fatty foods. The blunted response could lead to an increase in the need for rewarding foods (Wang et al. 2009). Currently it is unclear whether excessive eating increases the production of dopamine. The foods containing protein that form the building blocks of amino acid, including tyrosine, are essential for the production of dopamine.

This suggests that ingesting proteins boosts the levels of dopamine. Eating a high protein breakfast, to include eggs, lean meats and dairy products was less likely to reduce midmorning cravings whilst increasing dopamine levels (Hoertel et al. 2014). Taking meals at regular intervals will prevent sudden mood swings, regulate the appetite and reduce the temptation to overindulge.

Diets frequently recommend that the intake of starchy carbohydrates be restricted or avoided; however, they are important components of the diet as they promote stable blood glucose levels, which have a positive effect on the appetite. Bread, porridge, potatoes, and some fruits are high in carbohydrates, but providing their intake is limited, they will have the desired effect.

Everything in moderation is the key to a healthy diet, together with the knowledge of the influence that food has on the father's mental wellbeing. Some have experienced significant mood changes following moderation and consideration of their diet. The challenge to encourage the father to eat sensibly can be a daunting, particularly when faced with a man who has spent years indulging in a junk food diet, where a hamburger and a carton of chips satisfy instant hunger. The desire not to eat or not to be bothered to eat is strong, but equally not eating and gaining sufficient nutrients, is in itself a precursor to further depressive symptoms.

The mention of 'sensible eating' and dieting can be an anathema to some fathers who will see this as an impractical solution. Talk of quinoa, chia seeds and blueberries may cause abhorrence, particularly if budgets are tight. Introducing a diet that incorporates 'a healthy lifestyle' appears to be more acceptable. Simple substitution of brown bread sandwiches instead of white bread is doable. Curries made of nuts and vegetables rather than meats, smoothies instead of protein drinks are also doable. The solution is to eat small meals frequently, avoiding any temptation to eat foods high in sugar or fats, which immediately sate hunger, but to concentrate on the healthier fruit and vegetables.

For some it may be difficult to recall when and what they last ate, which is where a food diary is useful. The father can be encouraged to list everything eaten, when it is eaten, on a day-to-day basis. Eating habits differ from a weekday to a weekend, therefore completing the record from a Friday to Monday are probably the more important days. He will be able to visually record what he has consumed, not only at the present time but for future reference. The time is important to note when he felt he was most able to eat and the amount that he felt he was able to consume. This will help him to understand why he was eating more or less than usual and the reasons for the change in his dietary habits.

Sleep

The average amount of sleep required for an adult is seven to nine hours; however, constantly being tired is probably a sign of insufficient sleep. A satisfying night's sleep is a prerequisite for good physical and mental health. It has been postulated that the number of people presenting with insomnia has increased in recent years possibly because of the cultural and socioeconomic situations in which they have found themselves. It is accepted that the day after a night of sleep disturbance or deprivation, that concentration and mood would be affected with the father admitting that he would have been able to perform more effectively if he had been able to have a good night's sleep. However, it is now generally understood that the action of sleep not only has an effect on physiological factors but on cognitive abilities.

Insomnia, fractured sleep and diurnal variation in sleep patterns are common symptoms of depressive mood. The main problem is not being able to settle down and relax to sleep. The inability to maintain sleep throughout the night or waking early can initiate feelings of lethargy and fatigue, which may permeate throughout the day. Approximately one third of the general population has reported problems with sleep inefficiency, but only a small minority has the diagnosis of insomnia. Sleep disturbances are also connected with adverse childhood experiences and has been linked with poor sleep patterns in adulthood (Kajeepeta et al. 2015, Pennestri et al. 2015).

One study found that if around four months of age the infant is unsettled during the night, there was a risk that the father's depressive symptoms would increase. This culminated in poor personal sleep and increased anger at his own ability to have a good night's sleep (Cook et al. 2014).

Sleep deprivation is a feature of depression and the rates are significantly increased in major depression with almost all those suffering reporting some sleep disturbances (Salo et al. 2012). The causes of sleep deprivation are as yet not fully understood, although the complexities of both the psychological and physiological causes are to probably responsible. A traumatic or stressful situation may account for the inability to settle to sleep and but long-term sleep deprivation is often caused by the ruminating, pervasive thoughts, which tend to keep the mind and body awake. A vicious circle may be created, with the pervading fear that as bedtime approaches the father prophesises that he will be unable to sleep at night and predictably the cycle of sleep deprivation becomes toxic.

Poor sleep-awake patterns can be altered by the content of the diet as an alteration in the composition of the gut microbiomes, which are possibly associated with poor sleep and a lack of concentration. The gut-brain access is the two-way interaction between the gastrointestinal tract and the nervous system. It is increasingly thought that the gut microflora are responsible for a range of health factors, including anxiety and depression. It has also been suggested that there is an association between the gut microbiota and cognitive flexibility. Therefore, for fathers who consume a high fat diet, this may have alterations in the proinflammatory markers which are relevant to the sleep process of sleep (Kohsaka et al. 2007, Anderson et al. 2017).

As well as other factors, poor sleep patterns have implications for the immune system as well as other factors. It is well known that sleep patterns alter when an infection is present in the body. Animal studies have shown that interactions between immune signalling cytokines and the serotonin system are intensified during an infection and might explain why there are changes in sleep during an infection (Imeri & Opp 2009). During normal sleep the brain temperature drops with non-rapid eye movement (NREM) sleep and increases when the brain goes into rapid eye movement sleep. If a fever is present this situation changes and the NREM sleep is distorted whilst the REM sleep is inhibited. It is believed that the immune system accommodates the infectious nature of the fever by conserving the body's energy (Kueger 2008). In depressive illnesses there is tendency for both disturbed REM sleep and abnormal cytokine profiles. Where the insomnia is persistent this may induce inflammation, and amongst other factors can cause chronic stimulation and alteration of the HPA axis which has a role in the determination of depressive disorders (Balbo et al. 2010). The cytokines are involved in the regulation of sleep by influencing the release of neurotransmitters in the hypothalamus. This helps with the awake-sleep cycle.

One study found that there were increased levels of cortisol in insomniacs when compared with the normal levels. There were higher levels in the evening and during the first part of the night, which indicated that these are associated with the difficulties in sleep disturbances (Vgontzas et al. 2001). There may be a delay of between twelve and twenty-four hours in which the cortisol levels return to normal and in some cases of chronic sleep deprivation, the rate is slower than normal. The loss of sleep does not appear to be an acute stressor for the HPA axis but it does appear to affect the recovery time for the HPA response (Leproult et al. 1997). It was found that those who have been diagnosed with insomnia had evidence of a relationship between sleep and inflammation, with the levels of the proinflammatory cytokines being higher than in those with a healthy sleep pattern (Vgontzas et al. 2002).

The National Institute for General Medical Sciences describes the circadian rhythms as 'physical, mental, and behavioural changes that follow a daily cycle. They respond primarily to light and darkness in an organism's environment' (Circadian Rhythms, September 2017, p. 1). Hence they are responsible for the process of sleeping at night and being awake during the day. The circadian rhythms synchronise the sleep-awake behaviours, cellular function, hormone secretion and gene expression.

Problems occur when the process of sleep and preparation for sleep are disturbed, and the full circadian cycle cannot be completed. Photoreceptors within the eye are used to detect light and the exposure to natural sunlight, which has blue light, is detected by the retina. Melanopsin, a light-sensitive retinal protein, is expressed by photoreceptors, which respond most strongly to blue light. This signals the hypothalamus to produce cortisol and warm up the body. When darkness approaches the hypothalamus signals the production of the hormone melatonin, which is responsible for sleep and the body temperature drops. This sensitivity allows the circadian rhythm to be synchronised with the twenty-four-hour solar day.

Management of sleep problems

Sleep hygiene is important and a routine, if possible, at bedtime helps to induce sleep. Signals of tiredness are a good indicator to sleep, and making a habit of going to bed and waking up at the same time each day is recommended, although this might not always be possible because of the needs of a fractious infant. Taking a warm bath or shower prior to bedtime can help to lower the body temperature and induce sleep more quickly, or reading a book an hour before going to bed helps to relax the body in preparation for sleep.

The environment of the bedroom in important and ideally should be dark, cool and quiet with comfortable bedding. If this is not practical, in order to remedy this, blackout curtains, an eye mask and ear plugs may be useful additions to the night time routine, but as night time infant care has to be shared, making this possible presents its own challenges. Sometimes listening to voices or music on the radio can induce sleep, or help to return to sleep if there is sleep impairment.

It is tempting have a 'lie in' after a restless night, but the advice is to commit to regular night time routines, to enable the body's circadian clock to adjust. It is important to not to consume an excessive meal or to smoke prior to sleeping. The intake of caffeine in tea or coffee should be avoided for at least six hours before bedtime as these substances can induce anxiety and inhibit sleep. Drinking water during the day is recommended rather than later at night, to prevent having to wake to go to the bathroom during the night.

There are several relaxation techniques which the father can easily apply to lessen anxiety and improve sleep. These include mindfulness, yoga, meditation and breathing exercises. Practicing these techniques during the daytime can help to improve mood and act as a trigger to activate the relaxation techniques at night. The most common breathing exercises are to breathe in for the count of four, hold the breath for the count of five and breath out to the count of six. An alternative is to completely inhale into the tummy hold momentarily and release the air through the nose, as slowly as possible. Whatever the method, the principle is that controlling breathing by counting breaths influences the neuronal oscillations throughout the brain, particularly the amygdala.

Automatic breathing modulates the cingulate cortex whilst volitional pacing of the breath engages the frontotemporal-insular cortices (Herrero et al. 2018). The body is constantly in a state of equilibrium and achieves respiratory sinus arrhythmia. When inhaling, blood is drawn from the heart into the vasculature of the lungs. This depletes the rest of the body of normal blood flow, but it is compensated by an increase in the heart rate. When exhaling, the blood flow returns from the lungs and the heart rate decreases (Herrero et al. 2018).

There is increasing awareness on the impact of light emitted from televisions screens, phones, tablets and computers. The exposure to this blue light inhibits the production of melatonin which in turn affects the circadian rhythm.

There is now strong evidence to suggest that there is a relationship between sleep disruption and mood disorders. For some the anxiety may be so severe the difficulty in controlling it necessitates a pharmaceutical intervention. The severity of the disturbance in the mood has an association with the amount of sleep impairment. Therefore, treating the insomnia improves the mood state. The actions of the antidepressants are able to improve the quality of sleep; they also have a protective effect against sleep deprivation induced anxiety (Khazaie et al. 2010, 2013).

Evidence suggests that often, the preferred and more widely prescribed type of medication for insomnia and depression is trazadone, which has both antidepressive properties and sedative effects. It is a receptor antagonist and inhibits the serotonin reuptake. The actions of the drug improve the continuity of sleep but does not suppress REM sleep and promotes slow wave sleep. One dose at bedtime helps to improve the onset of and the quality sleep (Roth et al. 2011).

There has been some success in combining antidepressant medication with mindfulness- based cognitive behavioural therapy, which focuses primarily on the insomnia. Following treatment there was an improvement in the quality of sleep together with a reduction in anxiety and depressive symptoms (Yook et al. 2008).

However, turning off the phone and implementing some or all of the recommended techniques to solve insomnia are not always practical or manageable, and there may be more complex reasons for why the father may not be able to sleep. Telling, talking and treatment can help, but recognising the importance of sleep is the most essential component of good mental health.

Exercise

Exercise can lower both anxiety levels and depressive symptoms and improve the quality of sleep; however, the irony of depressive symptomology is the inability to be motivated to do any exercise. Although there is little known about the underlying mechanisms, a molecular link has been found between exercise and resistance to depression. Exercise induces expression of the transcriptional coactivator PGC-1a in muscle (Agudelo et al. 2014). A mechanism was identified by which skeletal muscle induced by exercise training changes tryptophan—kynurenine metabolism and protects from stress-induced depression. Tryptophan is converted to kynurenine and is linked to neuroinflammation, considered to be one of the causes of depression, thus explaining the beneficial effects of exercise for those with depressive symptomology. The suggestion is that moderate levels of activity for twenty–thirty minutes a day can also help to prevent depressive symptoms. There is significant evidence to demonstrate that physical activity can improve depressive symptoms (WHO 2010). One of the key benefits of being active is that it can reduce stress.

Exercise can mimic the action of stress as it requires increased blood flow, metabolism and other chemical reactions to restore the physiological processes. It has been found that exercise causes a heightened increase in the HPA axis activity. Although there have been several animal studies on the effect of exercise on the HPA axis, there have been very few studies in humans. Some have examined the effect of exercise on cortisol and ACTH. It is believed that moderate to excessive exercise elevates the cortisol levels. One study examined the response of depressed female adolescents to exercise and found the symptoms had diminished and their urinary cortisol levels had decreased (Nabkasorn et al. 2006). The more vigorous the exercise, the greater the changes in serotonin levels, suggesting that the impact of exercise on serotonin neurotransmission may depend on the exertion of the exercise. One study found that the combination of moderate and vigorous, aerobic and resistive exercise does appear to reduce symptoms of depression (Schoffstall & Barclay 2014). In studies, it was found that exercise compared favourably to antidepressant medications and improved the depressive symptoms when used in addition to medication. This was also found in comparisons with cognitive behavioural therapy (Carek et al. 2011).

Activities

Engaging in sport and physical activities partially encounter the same neurophysiological changes as antidepressants. The epinephrine activity is strengthened, which promotes cell growth in the brain and prevents the death of cells in the hippocampus. Together with these changes, sport and physical activity also lead to a reduced activity of cortisol, and therefore has an effect similar to psychotropic drugs. (Wegner et al. 2014).

Sport, as a means of engaging men, is becoming increasingly popular. As well as providing a platform for the opportunity to exercise, it also offers the context of related factors such as social support, activity, control, sharing, communicating and sharing as well as the ability to become self-efficient. Therefore this supports exercise as the presumed mechanism of change in the link between exercise and depressive symptoms (McArdle et al. 2012).

The addition of animals and their therapeutic value emphasises the inherent value of all organisms. Although the evidence for equine-assisted psychotherapy is limited, it is however, emerging as an innovative treatment for depression. It helps to rebuild communication skills. The horse's acute perception can detect anxiety; therefore, learning to have a calm approach can reduce the stress of both the horse and rider. It also focuses on the ability to read non-verbal cues, empathy and self- awareness (Lee et al. 2016). Together with horses, there is also support in the literature to suggest that canine assisted psychotherapy also has similar therapeutic benefits, including engagement and retention (Jones et al. 2016).

The high intensity sports of squash, rock climbing and skydiving all offer an adrenaline-filled experience but also have beneficial effects on anxiety and depressive symptoms. The precise hand-eye coordination of squash enables the mind to concentrate on the game and not on outside forces. Some have found this therapeutic and helped to relearn how to manage stress.

Boulder climbing is a method of rock climbing, but on the ground. In some areas it is prescribed for depression. Men who did this for three hours a week over eight weeks noted a reduction in their depressive symptoms (Luttenberger et al. 2014). One study has found that skydiving can improve mental health. Extreme sports trigger a range of positive experiential outcomes. The release of endorphins coupled with the ability to put emotions into perspective, has a therapeutic effect. The focus was not on risk-taking but the potential outcome of death following a mismanaged mistake or accident. There was detailed preparation to minimise any negative outcomes as the argument is made that some everyday events have a high risk (Brymer 2010).

Some areas are offering young people a series of surf lessons, on prescription. One-to-one support is provided both in and out of the water. The aim is to reduce the stigma of therapy but offer the therapeutic principles of coping and increasing confidence.

Football and similar sporting clubs are taking on the mantle of mental wellbeing and are starting groups specifically for the non- sportsman, who may have a desire to play but not the confidence. In many instances the emphasis is not on playing the game but creating the atmosphere of support and the opportunity to discuss and share whilst playing.

Story of a father with poor lifestyle choices

Joseph, a twenty-seven-year-old father of twins, had never been a great eater and had suffered bouts of depression for most of his teenage years. As a health professional he was aware his diet was poor, as rather than cook, he preferred to visit the fast food outlets on his way home from his work. When he started his new job and his girlfriend told him she was pregnant, Joseph began to find the work and his home life increasingly stressful. Joseph said "I was so stressed at work, when I eventually finished my duty, I found I did not have the appetite for any food.

I had snacked during the day but felt nauseous after a couple of mouthfuls. Although I did not vomit, my stomach was uncomfortable and painful. When the twins were born, their demands came first, so trying to sleep and eat were not my priorities. I was never a good sleeper but in recent years I had noticed I had poor sleep hygiene, frequently looking at my iPhone whilst in bed or turning on my computer to check on some statistics.

I realised I was losing weight, quite a lot of it, but could not persuade myself to eat. The only way I did eventually manage it, was to convince myself that if I did not eat then they would put a nasogastric tube down my throat and force me to take nutrients. That was the gamechanger. I would close my eyes and eat, convincing myself it was good for me. Then I thought, this is nonsense, I need to eat better than I do. Although tired, I bought some decent foods and actually had a sense of achievement when I managed to make some healthy, easily digested meals.

I thought it practical to think about my sleep patterns and recognised that I needed a decent night's sleep, so took measures to help me fall off to sleep more easily, it took sometime but mindfulness and breathing exercises seemed to work. My mood certainly improved and I now try to avoid those food outlets and only go there when I want a treat".

The effect of nature and the outdoors has a calming effect on mood and being encouraged to take a walk, run or bike ride in the local park or along the beach and concentrate on the surroundings can help pacify intrusive thoughts. At home or in work, taking the time to stand and walk rather than sit for long hours also has beneficial effects. The depressed brain may fight against this activity but thinking positively and ignoring any messages of defeat, will help to conquer feelings of hopelessness. The more enjoyable the activity, the more the brain will benefit.

Despite the facts and advantages of exercising, when feeling depressed or anxious it is often difficult to conceive of any physical activity. Therefore, it is important that the benefits of active movements are understood and that despite the obstacles of getting moving, it will help to shift the depressive mood. Consideration of exercise as something that is achievable is a positive. Any movement of the body can provide an emotional benefit. As with sporting activities, exercise is more pleasurable when it is shared and there is social interaction and teamwork.

Classes and groups can be more appealing than solitary exercising and a personal trainer or life coach can inspire confidence as well as monitor activity. If the trainer has a sound knowledge of the challenges of depressive symptoms then programmes can be tailored which prove non-threatening. Committing to a plan and setting a limit on the amount of time spent exercising can make it less overwhelming and more attainable. Starting with small, simple exercises before building up to the more strenuous types can help to develop confidence and more can be accomplished over time.

With modern technology it is now easier to record what is happening to the father, when it is happening and why. A paper diary is still useful but, apps have been developed for use on the iPhone or iPad to record the amount of exercise, when it happens and the reasons for it. This can be extended to a food, mood, snooze and booze diaries which record the dietary intake, indicate what his mood is, when it happened and why did it happen, and what were the causes. A record of the sleep regimes and amount of alcohol or substances consumed will provide the father with detailed information about his condition and the effects, enabling him to set targets and strategies which will aid his recovery.

Whilst the importance of diet, sleep and exercise are recognised as being preventative or curative factors in mental disorders and illness, sometimes the potential influence is not fully appreciated. The pathways between these lifestyle factors and the association with the physiology of the body and the impact on the brain are often not given the attention they require. The interesting features are that when depression occurs there are changes in the sleep patterns, diet and need to exercise, and yet if there are external reasons why there are changes in the sleep pattern, poor eating habits or inability to exercise, this can lead to an increase in depressive symptomology. A toxic cycle arises. A poor diet, disruptive sleep pattern and reduced physical activities influence and change the construction of neurochemicals, neurotransmitters, hormones and neuroactivity. Likewise, the opposite can happen when depression occurs.

References

Agudelo LZ, Femenía T, Orhan F et al. 2014. Skeletal muscle PGC-1α1 modulates kynurenine metabolism and mediates resilience to stress-induced depression. *Cell*, 159, pp. 33–34.

Anderson JR, Carroll I, Azcaearw-Peril MA, Rochette AD, Heinberg LJ, Peat C, Steffen K, Manderino LM, Mitchell J, Gunstad J. 2017. A preliminary examination of gut microbiota, sleep, and cognitive flexibility in healthy older adults. *Sleep Medicine*, 38, pp. 104–107.

Balbo M, Leproult R, Van Cauter E. 2010. Impact of sleep and its disturbances on the hypothalamic- adrenal-pituitary-adrenal access activity. *International Journal Endocrinology*, 2010, p. 759234.

Beezhold BL, Johnston CS. 2012. Restriction of meat, fish, and poultry in omnivores improves mood: A pilot randomized controlled trial. *Nutrition Journal*, 11, p. 9.

Brymer E. 2010. Risk taking in extreme sports: A phenomenological perspective. *Annals of Leisure Research*, 13(1), pp. 218–238.

Carek PJ, Laibstain SE, Carek SM. 2011. Exercise for the treatment of depression and anxiety. *International Journal of Psychiatry in Medicine*, 41, pp. 15–28.

Cepeda MS, Stang P, Makadia R. 2016. Depression is associated with high levels of C-Reactive protein and low levels of fractional exhaled nitric oxide: Results from the 2007–2012 national health and nutrition examination surveys. *Journal of Clinical Psyhiatry*, 77(12), pp. 1666–1671.

Cook F, Giallo R, Petrovic Z, Coe A, Seymour M, Cann W, Hiscock H. 2014. Associations between unsettled infant behaviour, paternal depressive symptoms and anger. *Frontiers in Perinatal Mental Health – Looking to the Future*. Marcé Society conference abstracts. Archives of Women's Mental Health. doi: 10.1007/s00737-019-00953-9.

Dimitrios P, Makedou K, Zormpa A, Karampola M, Ioannou A, Hitoglou-Makedou A. 2016. Are dietary intakes related to obesity in children? *Journal of Medical Sciences*, 4(2), pp. 194–199.

Ford PA, Jaceldo-Siegl, Lee JW, Youngberg W, Tonstad S. 2013. Intake of Mediterranean foods associated with positive affect and low negative affect. *Journal of Psychosomatic Research*, 74(2), p. 142.

German L, Kahana C, Rosenfeld V, Zabrowsky I, Wiezer Z, Fraser D, Shahar DR. 2011. Depressive symptoms are associated with food insufficiency and nutritional deficiencies in poor community – dwelling elderly people. *Journal of Nutrition, Health and Aging*, 15, pp. 3–8.

Goldney RD, Eckert KA, Hawthorne G, Taylor AW. 2010. Changes in the prevalence of major depression in an Australian community sample between 1998 and 2008. *Australian and New Zealand Journal of Psychiatry*, 44, pp. 901–910.

Hanley J. 2017. Revisiting the family mealtime. *Journal of Health Visiting*, 5(1), pp. 50–50, Last Word.

Herrero JL, Khuvis S, Yeagle E, Cerf M, Mehta AD. 2018. Breathing above the brain stem: Volitional control and attentional modulation in humans. *Journal of Neurophysiol*, 119(1), pp. 145–159.

Hoertel HA, Will MJ, Leidy HJ. 2014. A randomized crossover, pilot study examining the effects of a normal protein vs high protein breakfast on food cravings and reward signals in overweight/obese 'breakfast skipping', late-adolescent girls. *Nutrition Journal*, 13(80).

Hu F. 2018. Foods that fight inflammation. *Harvard Women's Health Watch*. Harvard Health Publishing. https://www.health.harvard.edu/staying-healthy/foods-that-fight-inflammation, accessed 19 November 2019.

Imeri L, Opp MR. 2009. How (and why) the immune system makes us sleep. *Nature Reviews Neuroscience*, 10(3), pp. 199–210.

Jones MG, Rice SM, Cotton SM. 2016. Incorporating animal-assisted therapy in mental health treatments for adolescents: A systematic review of canine assisted psychotherapy. *PLOS ONE*, 14(1), doi: 10.1371/journal.pone.0210761

Kajeepeta S, Gelaye B, Jackson CL, Williams MA. 2015. Adverse childhood experiences are associated with adult sleep disorders: A systematic review. *Sleep Medicine*, 16, pp. 320–333.

Khazaie H, Moradi M, Tahmasian M, Rezaein M, Dabiry S, Nikray R, Rezaie L, Younesi G, Schwebel DC. 2010. Insomnia treatment by olanzapine. Is sleep state misperception a psychotic disorder? *Neurosciences (Riyadh)*, 15(2), pp. 110–111.

Khazaie H, Rasoul M, Ghadami R, Knight DC, Emamian F, Tahmasian M. 2013. (Insomnia treatment in the third trimester of pregnancy reduces postpartum depression symptoms: A randomized clinical trial. *Psychiatry Research*, 20(3), pp. 901–905.

Kohsaka A, Akira K, Laposky AD et al. 2007. High-fat diet disrupts behavioral and molecular circadian rhythms in mice. *Cell Metabolism*, 6, pp. 414–421.

Kueger JM. 2008. The role of cytokines in sleep regulation. *Current Pharmaceutical Design*, 14(32), pp. 3408–3416.

Lee PT, Dakin E, McLure M. 2016. Narrative synthesis of equine-assisted psychotherapy literature: Current knowledge and future research directions. *Health and Social Care in the Community*, 3, pp. 225–246.

Leproult R, Copinschi G, Buxton O, Van Cauter E. 1997. Sleep loss sleep loss results in an elevation of cortisol levels the next evening. *American Sleep Disorders Association and Sleep Research Society*, 20(10), pp. 865–870.

Lopresti AL, Hood SD, Drummond PD. 2015. A review of lifestyle factors that contribute to important pathways associated with major depression: Diet, sleep and exercise. *Journal of Affective Disorders*, 148(1), pp. 12–27.

Luttenberger K, Stelzer EM, Forst S, Schopper M, Kornhuber J, Book S. 2014. Indoor rock climbing (bouldering) as a new treatment for depression: Study design of a waitlist-controlled randomized group pilot study and the first results. *BMC Psychiatry*, 15, p. 201.

Masana MF, Haro JM, Mariolis A et al. 2018. Mediterranean diet and depression among older individuals: The multinational MEDIS study. *Experimental Gerontology*, 110, pp. 67–72.

McArdle S, McGale N, Gaffney P. 2012. A qualitative exploration of men's experiences of an integrated exercise/CBT mental health promotion programme. *International Journal of Men's Health*, 11(3), pp. 240–257.

Monster B. 2018. Diet linked to mental health. *The Mercury*, 15(12).

Nabkasorn C, Miyai N, Sootmongkol A, Junprasert S, Yamamoto, H Arita M, Miyashita K. 2006. Effects of physical exercise on depression, neuroendocrine stress hormones and physiological fitness in adolescent females with depressive symptoms. *European Journal of Public Health*, 16, pp. 179–184.

Pennestri MH, Moss E, O'Donnell K et al. 2015. Establishment and consolidation of the sleep-wake cycle as a function of attachment pattern. *Attachment & Human Development*, 17(1), pp. 23–42.

Roth AJ, McCall WV, Liguori A. 2011. Cognitive, psychomotor and polysomnographic effects of trazodone in primary insomniacs. *Journal of Sleep Research*, 20(4), pp. 552–558.

Salo P, Oksanen T, Sjosten N, Penetti J, Virtanen M, Kivimaki M, Vahtera J. 2012. Insomnia symptoms as a predictor of incident treatment for depression: Prospective cohort study of 40,791 men and women. *Sleep Medicine*, 13(3), pp. 278–284.

Sanchez-Villegas A, Toledo E, De Irala J, Ruiz-Canela M, Pla-Vida JL, Martinez-Gonzalez MA. 2012. Fast-food and commercial baked goods consumption and the risk of depression. *Public Health Nutrition*, 15, pp. 424–432.

Schoffstall J, Barclay T. 2014. Pilot study: Effects of exercise on depression symptoms using levels of neurotransmitters and EEG as markers. *Medicine & Science in Sports & Exercise*, 46(5S), pp. 218–219.

Sublette ME, Ellis SP, Geant AL, Mann JJ. 2011. Meta-analysis of the effects of eicosapentaenoic acid (EPA) in clinical trials in depression. *Journal of Clinical Psychiatry*, 72, pp. 1577–1584.

Szabo M. 2013. Foodwork or foodplay? Men's domestic cooking, privilege and leisure. *Sociology*, 47(4), pp. 623–638.

Vgontzas AN, Bixler EO, Lin HM, Prolo P, Mastorakos G, Vela-Bueno A, Kales A, Chrousos GP. 2001. Chronic insomnia is associated with nyctohemeral activation of the hypothalamic–pituitary–adrenal axis: Clinical implications. *Journal of Clinical Endocrinology & Metabolism*, 86, pp. 3787–3794.

Vgontzas AN, Zoumakis M, Papanicolaou DA, Bixler EO, Prolo P, Lin HM, Vela-Bueno A, Kales A, Chrousos GP. 2002. Chronic insomnia is associated with a shift of interleukin-6 and tumor necrosis factor secretion from nighttime to daytime. *Metabolism*, 51, pp. 887–892.

Wang JC, Hinrichs AL, Stock H, Budde J, Allen R, Bertelsen S, Kwon JM, Wu W, Dick DM, Rice J, Jones K, Nurnberger JI, Tischfield J, Projesz B, Edenberg HJ, Hesselbrock V, Crowe R, Schuckit M, Begleiter H, Reich T, Goate AM, Bierut LJ. 2004. Evidence of common and specific genetic effects: association of the muscarinic acetylcholine receptor M2 (CHRM2) gene with alcohol dependence and major depressive syndrome. *Human Molecular Genetics*, 13(17), pp. 1903–1911.

Wegner M, Helmich I, Machado S, Nardi AE, Arias-Carrion O, Budde H. 2014. Effects of exercise on anxiety and depression disorders: Review of meta- analyses and neurobiological mechanisms. *CNS & Neurological Disorders – Drug Targets*, 13(6), p. 1002.

WHO. 2010. *Global Recommendations on Physical Activity for Health*, Geneva: WHO Press.

Yook K, Lee SH, Ryu M, Kim KH, Choi TK, Suh SY, Kim YW, Kim B, Kim MY, Kim MJ. 2008. Usefulness of mindfulness-based cognitive therapy for treating insomnia in patients with anxiety disorders: A pilot study. *Journal of Nervous and Mental Disease*, 196, pp. 501–503.

Chapter 9

Pharmaceutical interventions

Referral to the medical services should always be considered for psychopharmaceutical medications. Antidepressants may be prescribed for the more severe forms of depression and a combination of medication and therapy has positive results.

There are many misconceptions about taking mood stabilisers, antidepressants and anti-anxiety drugs, and many encompass the tales of Valium (a benzodiazepine) being called 'mummy's little helper' because of the calming and later addictive effects of the drug. There are also mistaken beliefs about antidepressants causing zombie like features and of 'taking away your soul', whereby all thought processes are numbed and the ability to think clearly disappears. There is also the myth that the action of the drugs induces long periods of lethargy and sleep.

For some fathers there is the acknowledgement that taking medication would be viewed as a sign of defeat, coupled with the anxiety instigated if it became common knowledge that they were taking a psychiatric drug. It is not unusual for some fathers to discontinue the treatment, primarily because they are unable to cope with the feelings of being out of control, more drowsy or lethargic than usual or they may acquiesce to family pressure to stop their reliance on drug therapy. However, there is overwhelming evidence that this is one of the best therapies and so there should be a concerted effort to support him to ensure the full course of medication is taken as once treatment has been discontinued without medical advice, there is evidence of relapse.

It is important that the father understands the consequences of not taking prescribed medication as the solution may often be to replace the antidepressants by self-medicating with alcohol or drugs, both of which are depressants. Thus, unless the medication is taken regularly the cycle of depression continues. The benefits of medication, however, outweigh the grief associated with the depression or anxiety.

Contrary to popular belief, modern medication is well tolerated and the effects, if there are any, are mild, compared with those experienced in previous years. Common side effects may include mild upset stomachs, headaches and dryness of the mouth. The length of time for the drugs to become effective and side effects of the drugs should always be a consideration when explaining the reasons for the prescription. The normal length of time for the antidepressant to start to be effective is from two to three weeks, and they should be taken for at least six to nine months. Following nine months there should be a revaluation of the symptoms. If the father is well and shows no signs of depression then the medication can be tapered off and eventually stopped. In all cases it would be wise to monitor the mental health of the father to ensure that he and his physician are aware of any potential relapse.

Antidepressants

Selective serotonin reuptake inhibitors (SSRIs) work because they alter the release of serotonin at the synapses which means that the serotonin signalling is adjusted throughout the brain. SSRIs and serotonin norepinephrine reuptake inhibitors (SNRI's) are known to increase their respective monoamine levels in the brain.

The SSRI is swallowed, enters the blood stream where it travels to the brain and onto the synapses. The SSRIs function by inhibiting the uptake of serotonin, which is responsible for the regulation of the mood, sleep and appetite. They work by increasing the amount of serotonin found in the synapses in the central nervous system. This occurs through the pre and post synaptic nerve endings which communicate with each other through the synapses.

Serotonin is found in the vesicles which are located in the pre-synaptic neuron and is released into the synapse, which it travels across. Serotonin binds with the post synaptic vessels and then continues to signal to the neuron post synaptically. When serotonin is released, it is also reabsorbed back into the post synaptic neurons. When the SSRI blocks the reuptake, there is an accumulation and therefore an increase in the amount of serotonin in the synapses. This accounts for the length of time SSRIs take to become affective, often from four–six weeks (Baudry et al. 2010).

Often antidepressants are demonised because they are thought to be habitual, but there is now evidence to suggest that those on antidepressants have higher levels of brain-derived neurotrophic factor (BDN) and this in turn enlarges the hippocampus, indicating antidepressants could have a protective effect.

Antidepressants may be prescribed for the more severe forms of depression, and many studies have shown that a combination of medication and therapy have positive results (Leung et al. 2001, Dobson et al. 2008, Cuijpers et al. 2013, Halle et al. 2015). The selective serotonin reuptake inhibitor (SSRI) fluoxetine, commonly known as Prozac, is one of the only antidepressants that is significantly more effective at reducing major depression after eight weeks.

Tricyclic and related antidepressant drugs (TCAs) and SSRIs are the two main groups of antidepressant drugs in common use. Tricyclic antidepressants were first introduced in 1959 and until the advent of the SSRI drugs were the most commonly used. The newer tricyclic and related drugs are generally less toxic and have modified side effects.

When used in the stipulated therapeutic doses, the range of tricyclic antidepressants can be effective in the treatment of major depression. The drug

Amitriptyline has been evaluated and produces a 50%–100% improvement, compared with a placebo. Low dose regimes are apparently less effective (Barbui & Hotopf 2001, Furukawa et al. 2002).

Treatment with tricyclic and related antidepressants produces a parallel reduction in anxiety and improves sleep. The more severe the depression, the better the response is to the treatment. In the majority of cases, major depression resolves with treatment, but around 12%–15% of men continue to be depressed for up to two years. It has been suggested that relapse after one year is also a serious possibility. This may occur even if the original depression was resolved. This necessitates continuing the medication, even after the symptoms have resolved.

Psychological treatments are the optimal first-line of treatment, but Fluoxetine is the best available pharmacological treatment for moderate-to-severe depression for those fathers who lack access to psychotherapy or have not responded to non-pharmacological interventions.

Side effects of antidepressants

There may be a wide range of sometimes unpleasant side effects, when taking antidepressants, of which the father should be made aware as some of them may be unexpected. The therapeutic time for any antidepressant treatment to work successfully is four–six weeks, which is often a surprise, and disappointment for some fathers who believe the effect should be instantaneous. Side effects may be acute and usually diminish after a few days. The most common is a dry mouth and sometimes feeling nauseous. It is unclear why antidepressants should cause dryness in the mouth, often accompanied by difficulty in swallowing. It is possible it is caused by the stimulation of the serotonin 3 receptors, located at the hypothalamus and the brain stem, which aggravates the gastrointestinal tract and the blockage of the cholinergic receptors.

Some fathers noted an increase in their appetite and as a consequence an unwanted weight gain. This may be caused by the blockage of the dopamine receptor, in the mesocortical pathway. One study found that those taking antidepressants were 21% more likely to gain weight than those not on antidepressants (Gafoor et al. 2018). However, it is difficult to ascertain whether the antidepressants are associated with weight gain or if it is caused by lifestyle choices. A further reason is that as the depression is lessened, weight gain occurs because the appetite has improved. The risks of gaining weight have to be balanced against not receiving any treatment for the depression. Further complications with weight gain are the risks of suffering from weight-related illnesses such as type 2 diabetes and hypertension.

In line with weight gain, is the difficulty with constipation, a common side effect of antidepressants. It is caused because the neurotransmitter acetylcholine is blocked, and as a result, the lubricating intestinal secretions are drier, whilst the muscular contractions which propel the waste matter through the digestive tract are slowed. This is also the case with the problems associated with micturition.

The inability to see clearly because of the blurring of vision is also a side effect of antidepressants, particularly the tricyclics. This may be accompanied by itching or gritty sensation in the eye. When the neurotransmitter receptor is blocked, it also causes the cessation of tear production and causes 'dry eye syndrome'. It usually subsides within a few weeks of the treatment. If the condition persists, medication can be used to lubricate the eye, or another antidepressant medication may be more suitable.

An unwelcome side effect is fatigue and drowsiness, which may be unexpected if the father was hoping to be rejuvenated. However, some antidepressants contain more of a stimulant than others, which may prove more beneficial.

Less talked about side effects are the lack or loss of libido which is common with antidepressants. These can include a loss of sexual desire or a change in the desire for sex, problems with arousal, erectile dysfunction, discomfort, dissatisfaction or decreased orgasms. The severity of sexual side effects depends on the individual and the specific type and dose of the antidepressant. For some, the sexual side effects are minor or may decrease as their bodies adjust to the medication. For others, sexual side effects continue to be problematic.

It should always be suggested that the medication be given time to work. This may take several weeks, during which time the sexual side effects might improve. It may be helpful to take the medication before engaging in any sexual activity, particularly if it is only taken once a day. If it becomes a problem it is worth discussing this with the general practitioner for advice on reducing the dosage or changing the antidepressant for one that has fewer side effects. Those medications with the lowest known rate of sexual side effects are Bupropion hydrochloride (Zyban) and Vilazodone.

Those antidepressants more likely to cause problems are the selective serotonin reuptake inhibitors (SSRIs), which include; Citalopram (Celexa), fluoxetine (Prozac), Paroxetine and Sertraline (Zoloft) The serotonin and norepinephrine reuptake inhibitors (SNRIs), one of which is Venlafaxine desvenlafaxine, can also affect sexual functioning. The tricyclic and tetracyclic antidepressants which consist of amitriptyline, nortriptyline and clomipramine can also be problematic and also included in the group are the monoamine oxidase inhibitors, (MAOIs), Isocarboxazid (Marplan), Phenelzine (Nardil) and Tranylcypromine (Parnate).

Mirtazapine, an atypical antidepressant, however, was associated most with the weight gain. Mirtazapine tends only to be prescribed to people who are unable to take other, more widely used, antidepressants as weight gain is known to be a common side effect of this drug. Consideration may be given to the addition of a second antidepressant or another type of medication, which can counter the side effects, for example, Sildenafil (Viagra).

However, there is overwhelming evidence that this is one of the better therapies and a concentrated effort is required to support the father to ensure the full course of medication is taken. Once treatment has been discontinued without medical advice, there may be evidence of relapse.

Antipsychotic drugs

These drugs are used for the manic episodes of bipolar disorder and severe depression. There are complex mechanisms of the role of dopamine in the development of psychosis, and it is thought the neurotransmitter dopamine plays a key role. It is argued that the unusual experiences and behaviours which are associated with psychosis are associated with the function of dopamine in the brain. There are four major pathways: the first is the mesolimbic pathway which mediates the symptoms of paranoia and hallucinations. The blockage of dopamine receptors here reduces the symptoms of delusions and hallucinations. The second, the mesocortical pathway, mediates the symptoms of withdrawal and loss of motivation. The blockage of the dopamine receptors can contribute to the lack of motivation and to an exacerbation of fatigue. The third, the nigrostriatal pathway controls movement whereby a blockage of the dopamine receptor may cause excess movements. The last pathway is the tuberoinfundibular pathway which controls the secretion of prolactin. The blockage of the dopamine receptor in this pathway can result in high levels of prolactin in the blood, which can lead to sexual dysfunction (Kapur & Remington 2001).

Antipsychotic drugs are classified into first, typical, and second generation, atypical drugs. They block the D2 receptors. The first generation includes high potency drugs which include haloperidol, fluphenazine and trifluoperazine. These are heavy duty and therefore lower doses of medication are required. However, they may be responsible for sexual dysfunction and tremors. Some typical drugs have a lower potency, as an example chlorpromazine. In contrast to the first-generation drugs, second-generation antipsychotics block both the D2 receptors and the serotonin receptors. Serotonin inhibits dopamine release into the blocked serotonin receptors and may increase dopamine levels within the brain, where it is needed. Atypical antipsychotics briefly occupy the receptors allowing for normal dopamine transmission. This reduces the number of side effects compared to the first-generation drugs, depending on the drug's profile. Olazipine and clozapine can contribute to weight gain, whereas risperidone has the highest potential to contribute to fatigue and hypotension.

Medication for anxiety

Anxiolytics and sedatives are usually prescribed for anxiety and panic attacks. The release of gamma aminobutyric acid (GABA) has a calming and sedative affect. The muscles relax and the breathing slows. There are two main classes of anti-anxiety drugs. The class of drugs known as the benzodiazepines work on the GABA receptor, which is a neurotransmitter. The drug increases the frequency at which the GABA channels open and enhances the inhibitory action of GABA in the limbic system and slows down the depressive actions in some parts of the brain. The GABA receptors, which bind with the benzodiazepine, are also known as benzodiazepine receptors. When these attach to the GABA receptor it opens up negatively charged chloride ions meaning the neuron is less likely to fire a potential action.

All of the preparatory benzodiazepine medication on the market has the letters AZE contained within them. For example, drugs termed; Lorazepam, diazepam and temazepam. Most of the properties of these drugs are similar, with equally complicated neurotransmitter profiles.

Side effects of anti-anxiety medication

Prolonged use should be avoided as often there may be a tendency to be reliant on the effects of the medication and create dependence. Therefore, it is important to be vigilant when monitoring the prescribed course of the medication. Equally the drug should not be withdrawn abruptly as that can also lead to further complications. It may be difficult to secure the correct dosage, but successful management will help the father to understand the degree to which his emotions can be controlled and his anxiety blunted.

There has been a small minority of cases where an increase has been noted in the fathers' hostile and aggressive behaviour after taking benzodiazepines. Some have reported being overly garrulous and excited, too aggressive and making impulsive antisocial acts. However, adjusting the dose of the medication has been found to remedy the situation. The most common side effects present as nausea and mild stomach upsets. Some have reported a decrease in their attentiveness and ability to concentrate. Sleep disorders have been present with drowsiness and some muscle weakness. There have also been reports of vertigo, vision disorders and tremors. The more common side effects can result in agitation with some abnormal behaviour. There have been urinary disorders and a lack of libido. Very rare side effects are blood disorders, jaundice and psychosis (BNF 2015).

Treatment and management of specific disorders

Self-harm

It is often difficult for the father to admit to self-harming. It is important not to focus on the specific injuries or self-harming behaviours but to concentrate on what they are feeling and the thoughts they are experiencing. It can be easy to be shocked or disgusted by some self-harming behaviours, and the father is aware of this. Being non-judgemental is important, as any negative reaction can cause the father to withdraw and stop the discussion. Ultimatums should be avoided as it is natural to suggest they stop the harm otherwise they will seriously damage themselves. It has been found that this advice rarely works and may cause the father to be more surreptitious in his future behaviours (Garner 2001, NICE 2005).

Self-harm is not necessarily a chronic condition but can be resolved once the father feels he is able to discuss it and look for other solutions. Several successful pointers have been suggested as distraction techniques and include finding a safe space and having a resource that helps to keep him safe. This can be on an iPhone or iPad, collecting folders of photographs of family and happy occasions, saving funny comments that caused laughter, keeping cheerful videos and texts from trusted friends, which can be referred to when emotional feelings are overwhelming.

There are several ways in which the attention to self-harm can be diverted and can include concentrating on a film on YouTube, texting or reading. Lists of friends and family who have given permission to be woken up at 3 am to talk, a time when the father is most vulnerable is also a useful resource. Should the need to self-harm be overwhelming there are several strategies which may stop actual bodily harm. Placing ice cubes on the skin, plucking arm hairs or cracking knuckles creates pain, but the damage is minimal.

It is optimistic to believe that the father will stop his hurting behaviour once he receives help. This will take time and in the meantime damage limitation is possible. If the habit of cutting is persistent then using a clean blade is preferable. Where possible, to reduce the possibility of infection, it should be sterilised and never shared with others. Usage of the same implement for cutting will blunt over time, so changing them regularly will ensure cleaner cuts. A knowledge of first aid and accessible first aid kit containing plasters, bandages, antiseptic cream is useful.

A sound knowledge of their body structure is important in order to control the incidence of more serious injury, and having an understanding about what areas are more or least likely to bleed, or what wounds will probably heal more rapidly. Having an awareness of the pressure points and the force needed, helps to lessen the risk of haemorrhage. Recognising the impact any hurt or pain has on the body, and the way in which it reacts to external stimuli, is important. This, together with the need to allow for healing time can help to maximise safety and support the healing process both physically and mentally.

If the abuse involves eating disorders, then being acquainted with the action of excessive types of food and the impact on the digestive system can help to redress dietary habits. Drug misuse requires information on the action of illicit drugs and the effect of irreparable organ damage coupled with mental problems, caused by mixing different types of drugs. The influence of drugs and alcohol has been documented as have depressants, which lower brain activity and can increase feelings of stress and anxiety. Therefore, avoidance of consuming large quantities of alcohol should be encouraged, particularly in self-harm, as these can also lower inhibitions making self-harm more likely. Avoidance of drinking alcohol and taking drugs simultaneously prevents the danger of overdosing, with the unintended consequences.

Rewind therapy: Treating post-traumatic stress disorder

Sensations associated with a threatening situation are passed through the amygdala and formed in the sensory memory; this is passed to the hippocampus and from there to the neocortex. Here it is interpreted and stored as a verbal or narrative memory. The overload of a traumatic, life threatening incident means the sensory memories are kept within the amygdala and not passed onto the neocortex where they can be processed. Thus, the memory is not sufficiently processed, to enable it to have meaning, which means that it will be re-experienced in the form of flashbacks or panic attacks.

Rewind therapy works by allowing the traumatic memory to be reprocessed. This allows the incident to be stored as a non-threatening memory, albeit unpleasant rather than one that activates a terror response (Griffin & Tyrrell 2001). The technique works because the memory is transferred from the amygdala to the neocortex. The rewind technique allows the sensory memory to be reformulated and the enormity of the trauma put into perspective.

This allows the father to have control over what he chooses to experience and he does not have to share the intimate details of the therapy. It is known to be an effective and safe treatment. However, this should only be performed by an experienced and trained practitioner. This involves a relaxation technique which allows the father to be in a state of deep relaxation. The traumatic experience is allowed to resurface as they are asked to imagine a place where they feel safe and are at complete ease. In deep relaxed state the father is asked to imagine that they have a television with a remote control. They are asked to imagine floating to one side out of the body and to watch themselves, watching the screen, but not seeing the picture. The event is 'replayed' on the imaginary screen which starts with the beginning of the film and concludes when they feel safe. In the father's imagination they are asked to float back into their body and experience themselves going backwards through the trauma from where they felt safe, to where they feel safe. The event is watched again but this time in fast forward. These are repeated until there is no emotion felt when viewing the scenes (Guy & Guy 2003).

Treatment for OCD

One of the most common compulsions is hand washing with fathers attempting to clean their hands several times, unconvinced that they have removed all the debris. Therapy suggests that they should acknowledge that this is due to a faulty circuit in the brain and that nothing terrible will happen if they do not repeat the process. The father has to manually 'shift' the nucleus function to make it work by distraction therapy, which involves occupying their minds with other tasks. There is the risk that the compulsion is so overwhelming that they cannot resist but to acquiesce, but if they do, they should restrict the time and gradually reduce the amount of time spent doing the action. This requires practice until it becomes an automatic reaction to identify the compulsion and move onto another action, causing the brain to gradually become reprogrammed. It has been successfully demonstrated that by changing behaviour the brain can be changed.

Whatever the choice of therapy or treatment, the effectiveness is not immediate and for some fathers and some health practitioners this can be difficult to accept.

It is imperative to understand the importance of patience and not having immediate high expectations, but allowing the treatment to take its course. This will, in turn, help the father to understand the process of the condition, enabling him to recognise any potential early symptoms or reoccurrence in the future.

References

Barbui C, Hotopf M. 2001. Amitriptyline v. the rest: Still the leading antidepressant after 40 years of randomised controlled trials. *The British Journal of Psychiatry*, 178, pp. 129–144.

Baudry A, Mouillet-Richard S, Schneider B, Launay JM, Kellermann O. 2010. miR-16 targets the serotonin transporter: A new facet for adaptive responses to antidepressants. *Science*, 329(5998), pp. 1537–1541.

BNF. 2015. NICE guidelines for benzodiazepine (on-line). https://bnf.nice.org.uk

Cuijpers P, Sijbrandij M, Koole SL et al. 2013. The efficacy of psychotherapy and pharmacotherapy in treating depressive and anxiety disorders: A meta-analysis of direct comparisons. *World Psychiatry*, 12, pp. 137–148.

Dobson KS, Hollon SD, Dimidjian S et al. 2008. Randomized trial of behavioral activation, cognitive therapy, and antidepressant medication in the prevention of relapse and recurrence in major depression. *Journal of Consulting and Clinical Psychology*, 76, pp. 468–477.

Furukawa AT, McGuire H, Barbui C. 2002. Meta-analysis of effects and side-effects of low dosage tricyclics antidepressants in depression: Systematic review. *British Medical Journal*, 325, pp. 991–995.

Gafoor R, Booth HP, Gulliford MC. 2018. Antidepressant utilisation and incidence of weight gain during 10 years follow up population-based cohort study. *British Medical Journal*, 361, p. k1951.

Garner F. 2001. *Self Harm: A Psychotherapeutic Approach*. Hove: Brunner Routledge.

Griffin J, Tyrrell I. 2001. *The Shackled Brain: How to Release Locked-in Patterns of Trauma*. East Sussex: HG Publishing.

Guy K, Guy N. 2003. The fast way to cure trauma symptoms. *Human Givens Journal*, 9(4).

Halle RA, Gartlehner G, Gaynes BN et al. 2015. Comparative benefits and harms of second-generation antidepressants and cognitive behavioral therapies in initial treatment of major depressive disorder: Systematic review and meta-analysis. *British Medical Journal*, 351, p. h6019.

Kapur S, Remington G. 2001. Dopamine D2 receptors and their role in atypical antipsychotic action: Still necessary and may even be sufficient. *Biological Psychiatry*, 50(11), pp. 873–883.

Leung WC, Thornett AM, Curtis D, Chilvers C, Dewey M. 2001. Antidepressants and counselling for major depression in primary care. *British Medical Journal*, 323(7307), p. 282.

National Institute for Health and Clinical Excellence. 2005. The Management of depression. *BMJ*, 330(7486), pp. 267–268.

Chapter 10

Conclusion

Approaches towards fathers' mental health should differ from those directed towards mothers. The more sensitive caring approach should be avoided, focussing more on goals and planning his recovery. Times have changed. When men worked side by side in the mines, factories and farms they could talk, debrief and take advantage of the support networks. When they went to the pub for a pint after work they could reminisce and ruminate with friends. This is not so easy to achieve in the modern work office spaces or as the number of public houses decline. This is a part of wider global trend of involved fatherhood and a worldwide policy that recognised the contribution of fathers. Fathers want to be recognised as important and competent advocates for their partners' and their infants' care, both mentally and physically (UN 2011).

Raising awareness

Currently there are many campaigns addressing the needs of fathers and some are directed specifically at fathers' mental health (Fathers Reaching Out, iHV). The emphasis is on the importance of mental health during the perinatal period for not only the mother and infant, but the father too. Studies have demonstrated the impact poor mental health can have on a father and his relationship with his infant and family, but have also demonstrated how low mood and anxiety can be ameliorated with correct support and guidance. Fathers now play a prominent role in child care and their needs must not be marginalised.

The facts confirm that fathers can be influenced by anxiety and depression in utero, if their mother has suffered from a mood disorder or mental illness. Often this translates into the father sometimes suffering from a mental illness during this childhood, adolescence or early adult life. These can present in various forms to include bipolar disorder, psychosis, schizophrenia, autistic spectrum disorder and post-traumatic stress disorder during the postnatal period. This, as the evidence shows, brings challenges and questions. It is the responsibility of society to meet those challenges and answer the questions.

Information

The stigma of mental illness makes it difficult for men to address some of the issues that makes them question their parenting and intimate relationship abilities. In the first instance, talking with fathers has opened up interesting perspectives. Fathers do want information. They don't want it dressed up in sensitive or academic language. They want it straight, direct, factual, specific and focussed on that which resonates with their experience of life. They determine the need for more father-friendly promotional materials, from sources currently dominated by mother-friendly issues (Sherriff & Hall 2011, Baldwin & Bick 2018).

As an example, the provision of visual material in the form of photographs and drawings which demonstrate the involvement of the real father in the breastfeeding process (Brown & Davies 2014). Pictures that are not posed, depicting the 'ideal scenario', but real photos demonstrating real emotions in the real world. A regular journal supplement or leaflet, targeted exclusively at fathers would make them feel more inclusive. Data on child care and the impact of fathering, specifically detailing how the impact of their emotions and that of their infant have mutual benefits, and ways in which these can be achieved should be readily available.

This need not be confined to breastfeeding but could be expanded to encompass all aspects of infant and child development, including in utero. Areas that could be further explored include the importance of chronic stress on the parents, foetus and infant, and the need to avoid, or minimise stressful situations. This includes understanding the impact of financial difficulties and domestic abuse and the influence lifestyle choices have on mental wellbeing, the reciprocal joy of having emotional attachment with the mother and infant and the foibles of intimate relationships and sex.

Literature for fathers on mental disorders and illness is sparse. The availability of pamphlets on all of the disorders are scarce making it difficult to discreetly secure a leaflet from a clinic or health centre, if any were available. The growth of internet platforms has increased with the escalation of the engagement of pregnant and new mothers. These sites provide a venue for women to express and share thoughts on parenting and to offer solutions to each other. Some sites welcome the input of fathers and are currently aimed at parents, rather than single genders (Salzmann-Erikson & Eriksson 2013). There are excellent websites with copious information but often the father has no inclination to access them unless he needs help because he feels he is suffering, making him responsible for his own health.

A recent furore happened when a celebrity was pictured carrying his infant in a papoose. He was ridiculed in some media quarters for being emasculated. However, this was revoked by a backlash of other men who suggested that there must be uncertainty about one's own masculinity to be concerned with how another man carries his child. Nevertheless, this unhelpful tirade only deepens the gap between the role of parents.

Health professionals

Fathers would like more recognition of their role by health professionals and not confined to back rooms or told to go to the pub when issues around their partner's and infant's wellbeing are being discussed. Fathers need support, too, and it should be the remit of any health professional to ensure that the father's mental health is good and if it is not, then what resources are available to support the father. This can be achieved in the same way as the mother's mental health is assessed, and it has been advocated that this assessment should be universal (Austin et al. 2013). Taking a blood pressure is often seen as mandatory, so should an assessment of mental health – acknowledging the constraints of not being able to diagnose many mental illnesses by a physical examination.

Access to a health professional, however, may be difficult because fathers often return to work following the birth although in recent years paternity leave has made access easier. Historically fathers have not been invited to baby clinics and child development appointments. This is changing, but some fathers remain difficult to access. However, with sufficient notice of an impending visit by a health professional or attendance required at a clinic, the father should be able to make the necessary arrangements to attend (Baldwin et al. 2018).

The lived experiences from fathers who have coped with the difficulties of their own anxieties and depression have helped fathers to understand and relate to how others are feeling and coping with life. However, fathers are usually less likely to attend postnatal groups or other organised activities specifically designed for mothers. It has been proposed that separate antenatal and breastfeeding classes are required for both genders. As this is an innovative, developing area this will enable fathers to acquire and widen their own requirements for group interactions.

Despite all of the obvious symptoms presented, they are often missed or misinterpreted, because why would men become depressed? Surely that is the domain and privilege of the mother who carried and gave birth to the infant. The time to recognise paternal depression has come. However, fathers still present at health centres with somatic aches and pains of unknown origin, as often that is the most acceptable reason to visit the doctor. Exploring all of the facets of depression, and as it is presented should lead to a diagnosis of paternal depression. Perhaps it will. Prevention is better than cure and being aware of the risk factors, presentation of symptoms and the routes to access care are vital to help keep fathers healthy, both physically and mentally.

Record keeping

The emphasis has been and is on the mother's mental health and as a result the mental of health of the father is often excluded, ignored or marginalised. Testimony to this is the record keeping of health professionals who will often store copious records of the mother's health, but little relating to that of the father.

In some cases, there is little reference to the father's mental health following the initial months post birth. There is a growing emphasis to change records to ensure the there is a note made of whether the father was present when either attending a clinic or being visited by a health practitioner. Where these data have been captured it appears that the ratio of mothers to fathers is 4:1 (Price 2018). The wording of any correspondence and literature is often directed at the mother, inviting her and her infant to clinics, and informing her of infant care.

An awareness of the conditions and their process can allow mothers and fathers to have the confidence to confide and sometime confess how they feel. This knowledge is a privilege and helps the parents to understand themselves.

Limitations of the health practitioner

It is important to understand the limitations of the role of the health practitioner in helping the depressed father, and knowing when to refer onto another speciality or support service. There is no one size fits all and sometimes health practitioners can feel impotent if there is no significant progress or improvement. It is essential to understand the process of the father's condition and that perhaps a deeper, more intense therapeutic approach from another source is more appropriate, particularly if there is a threat of suicide. Referral should never be seen as a failure but a skill.

The are many reasons for referring the father onto a general practitioner, psychiatrist, specialist perinatal mental health team and/or social services. These include the father expressing thoughts about self-harming, taking his own life, or that of his partner or his infant, admitting to ongoing domestic violence and violence.

It is sometimes difficult to support fathers that need help. The reasons may be through inexperience or preference. If it is through inexperience, then discussion with a mentor or supervisor should ensure the health practitioner has the ability, skills and confidence to undertake the task. Talking comes naturally to most, but active listening is a skill. However, it is only with practice and patience that it will become easier. The fact is that some health practitioners have a fear of mental illness and believe it is the remit of other professionals yet it is quite clearly everyone's business to ensure that mothers, fathers and their families have the best possible mental health.

There might be a time when the therapeutic interventions do not appear to be progressing, the situation has stabilised and it is taking longer than anticipated. Most therapeutic interventions suggest the sessions are no longer than six weeks. If that point has been reached, then with mutual agreement, the father should be referred to another organisation or therapist. Some fathers may have entrenched problems that, even with the support from the most experienced practitioners, they are unable to extricate themselves from it. A fresh perspective, from another source of specialised therapy may help them to assimilate and challenge their emotions. The father will have lived with his condition for a long time, and probably feels some respite from any intervention, so waiting for an appointment will not be demanding.

An increasing number of midwives are also trained in perinatal mental health and illness and general practitioners are able to access substantial training. The community psychiatric teams have long been aware of the needs of mothers and fathers during the perinatal period and have been able to treat them accordingly, but as awareness grows it is hoped the management will be 'Everyone's Business' (MMHA).

Helping the partner to understand

Living with someone who is suffering from a mood disorder, albeit anxiety or depression can be debilitating for the partner. Often, they are the first to notice the mood changes but sometimes the last to seek help. It is important to ensure that the partner is aware of the process and progression of the disorder. Health practitioners are not available twenty-four hours a day, and therefore the partner has an important role to play. The mother of a new-born infant has enough to preoccupy her and may feel resentful when she feels unsupported at the time she needs it most. It is pertinent to be able to advise the partner how to both manage and support the father's condition.

The partner should be strongly advised against suggesting that it is not unusual for him to feel like this, as it is probably a phase he is going through, which most other fathers experience. That he doesn't look depressed and she knows exactly how he feels as she feels the same. He can manage this alone and should man up, what has he got to be depressed about? He does not need any help from anyone, especially the health visitor or psychiatrist. It is all in his head and he needs to be more positive. Blaming him and implying it is his own fault as he also wanted a baby, is also unhelpful.

A more positive approach is to recognise the father is suffering and that he probably feels dreadful; however, it is possible to feel like that and still be a good father. Making mistakes, being out of control and not being able to respond appropriately are part of the condition, but that is okay. Whatever help he decides to access is the proper course of action, taking medication, going to therapy and or speaking with friends. He will get better.

The level of the depression may be such, that the sense of any low mood or disinterest may jeopardise the father's interactions with the pregnancy. He may withdraw or isolate himself from social settings and some of his perceived responsibilities. If his partner or the health practitioner is aware of his mental health history, this will be the time to consider him being prescribed medication to help him cope with the ensuing pressures.

The problem of over one in three men not knowing how to help a friend who is suffering and having a tough time, has been highlighted by one television channel (Dave 2019) who has partnered with the organisation CALM to simply say: 'Be the mate you would want by texting phoning or tweeting'. This encourages fathers to not be afraid to ask how their mates are feeling by suggesting they check out how they are feeling and if they need any help.

In 2015 men were considered to have the right to be involved and have equal share in child care and as a result the UK government agreed to introduce shared parental leave. However, recent statistics put the number of men taking up this opportunity as just 1%. This raises the question of why this is the case, and how men feel about this change to their ideas of inspirational masculinity. There is the assumption that all men are working whereas there are areas within the UK where a substantial number of men are unemployed and are at the home at all times. However, anecdotal evidence suggests that some of these fathers resume the role of the traditional father and leave the child care to the mother.

Family communication

Spending a significant amount of time on social media is now the norm. Children indulge in solitary screen time instead of partaking and interacting in hobbies and sports. Parents who are equally absorbed in the screen ignore their children's cues for attention. Children as young as eighteen months are seen watching iPad screens. Within less than thirty seconds, social media and Instagram allow instant access to the world and its news. Whereas this has great advantages it also means that access is mostly unfiltered and can have damaging consequences. The posts, which convey the contented father, providing all the needs of his family, can resonate badly with the father who is financially compromised. There is increasing evidence that cyberbullying is growing, and this has impacted on self-esteem and mental health significantly. There seems to be a compulsion to look at the screen and to read comments, no matter how hurtful or detrimental. It is a case of having the knowledge but also the wisdom to understand what is happening.

Socialising with the family is rapidly diminishing, unless it is on high days, holidays and birthdays. The fantasy of the traditional Christmas dinner is often portrayed by the media during the festive season, yet the traditional meal eaten around the table is no longer the norm. The interior design programmes certainly determine the status of the dining room as an essential part of everyday life. However, how often is it used for meals as opposed to a work or play station? It was a place of cohesion, to share experiences and discuss the day's events. There were rites about who sat where, the father at the head and rituals which involved hand washing prior to eating, prayer before the meal, table manners, which involved eating with the correct cutlery. The meat was the only joint on the table, wrists and elbows were not acceptable. There was the expectation that the choice of meal presented suited everyone. Permission was sought to talk and to leave the table.

The table is a stable place to meet and eat and previously, has served humanity well. Mealtimes offer children the opportunity to talk with their parents and siblings and an occasion to bond and share the events of the day. It is a time to destress, gauge opinions, listen and discuss common goals and themes, understand the ground rules and why they are important. There is time and space for the family to bond, connect and attach. If the media is still able to sell the fantasy, then perhaps it is still feasible to eat around a table.

Preventative measures in school

Mental health measures should be a familiar tool within the school curriculum, ensuring that school leaders are aware of mental wellbeing amongst their pupils. This cannot be achieved without sufficient training, and therefore this should be a priority and appropriately resourced. Teachers often argue they are there to teach and not be responsible for the social upbringing of the child; however, there is now a sea change, with both teachers and parents recognising the increased pressure of poor concentration and social skills that can impact the learning capability of the child. Teachers, often like the children, have a need to understand how to retain, maintain a healthy lifestyle and to stay well. Techniques, such as relaxation and mindfulness, or as is becoming increasingly popular, poetry reading, once brought into the classroom can provide a toolkit for life, on managing any anxiety, the child may encounter. Peer support programmes on mental health can help youngsters to care for each other. They could be encouraged to understand how feelings can affect thoughts, and these can dictate how that child may react and why he reacts as he does. This greater understanding can be reinforced by experts in mental health, situated within the school, whose availability will allow pupils to talk whenever they feel vulnerable, anxious or alone. This unconscious persuasion of the mind will help to re programme unhealthy behaviours.

The father

The most important factor in father's mental health is recognition—recognition of the facts that the father may be anxious, depressed, manic, psychotic, bipolar and everything in between. The father's behavior is probably the best indicator and any deviation from the norm should be a signal that things are 'not right'. Having established that the father is 'unwell' the next step is to talk with him and together decide the best course of action or type of management of the situation that suits him.

There are a growing number of organisations, statutory and third sector, dedicated to fathers with mental health problems. There are specialists in perinatal mental health who can advise on the condition and as necessary, treat and manage cases. There are also statutory and voluntary organisations that specialise in helping mothers, fathers and their families and would welcome the opportunity to share their knowledge.

Previous generations of fathers were denied the luxury of recognition, assessment, management and treatment; they had to suffer the terrible consequences of their disabling mental disorders and illnesses. How different their lives would have been if they had been afforded help and support. However, there remains a long way to go in the battle to conquer mental illness. Campaigns have been partially successful in addressing the needs of fathers, but policies and protocols have to change, enabling paternal anxiety and depression to be at the forefront of services for the sake of the mental health of future generations.

References

Austin M, Hanley J, Wisner K. 2014. Marcé international Society position statement on psychosocial assessment and depression screening in perinatal women. *Best Practice Research Clinical Obstetric Gynaecology*, 28(1), pp. 179–187.

Baldwin S, Bick D. 2018. Mental health of first time fathers – it's time to put evidence into practice. *JBI Sumari*, 16(11), pp. 2064–2065.

Baldwin S, Malone M, Sandall J, Bick D. 2018. Mental health and wellbeing during the transition to fatherhood: A systematic review of first time fathers' experiences. *JBI Database of Systematic Reviews and Implementation Reports*, 16(11), pp. 2118–2191.

Brown A, Davies R. 2014. Fathers' experiences of supporting breastfeeding: Challenges for breastfeeding promotion and education. *Maternal and Child Nutrition*, 10(4), pp. 510–526.

Dave. 2019. Partnered with campaign against living miserably. https://corporate.uktv.co.uk/news/article/dave-starts-conversations-against-living-miserably-new-podcast/

Price R. 2018. A project to support fathers with paternal depression. *Journal of Health Visiting*, 6(8), pp. 380–386.

Salzman-Erikson M, Eriksson H. 2013. Fathers sharing about early parental support in health care-virtual discussions on an internet forum. *Health and Social Care in the Community*, 21(4), pp. 381–390.

Sherriff N, Hall V. 2011. Engaging and supporting fathers to promote breastfeeding: A new role for health visitors? *Scandinavian Journal of Caring Sciences*, 25, pp. 467–475.

United Nations. 2011. Men in Families and Family Policy in a Changing World. United Nations, New York: Department of Economic and Social Affairs.

Index

Printed in Great Britain
by Amazon

50805262R00090